CW01391150

'We are born loveable and peaceable as you say... But
boy does that get screwed up along the way.'
Dr Cathy Wield, Author and Specialist Emergency Medicine Physician

'A cracking read.'
Tim Newell, former Governor HM Prison Grendon

'I've just finished your incredible book—bloomin 'eck!'
Erwin James, Guardian Correspondent

'Original and authentic.'
Dave Marteau, former Head, HM Prisons Drug Addiction Service

'Your work will certainly help many to eventually come out of
their inner emotional prison...to live freely and responsibly.'
Alice Miller, Therapist

'What Bob achieved was magical, he helped so many...'
Charles Bronson

'I can't recall coming across anything like these
insights from any other doctor, psychiatrist, psychologist, analyst, scientist, academic or philosopher.'
Dr Clive Sherlock, Consultant Psychiatrist, Adaptation Practice, Oxford

Friendless Childhoods Explain War

Copyright © 2023 Dr Bob Johnson.

All intellectual property and associated rights are hereby asserted and reserved
by the author in full compliance with UK and international law. No part
of this book may be copied, reproduced, stored in any retrieval system or
transmitted in any form or by any means without the prior written permission
of the publishers to whom all such rights have been assigned worldwide.

The Foreword is the copyright of Martin Brunt.

ISBN 978-1-914603-39-6 (Paperback)
ISBN 978-1-914603-40-2 (EPUB ebook)
ISBN 978-1-914603-41-9 (PDF ebook)

Published 2023 by Waterside Press Ltd
www.WatersidePress.co.uk

A catalogue record for this book can be obtained from the British Library.

Ebook *Friendless Childhoods Explain War* is available as
an ebook including through library models.

Printed and bound by Severn, Gloucester, UK.

Friendless Childhoods Explain War

Dr Bob Johnson

Foreword Martin Brunt

❧ WATERSIDE PRESS

Contents

About the author

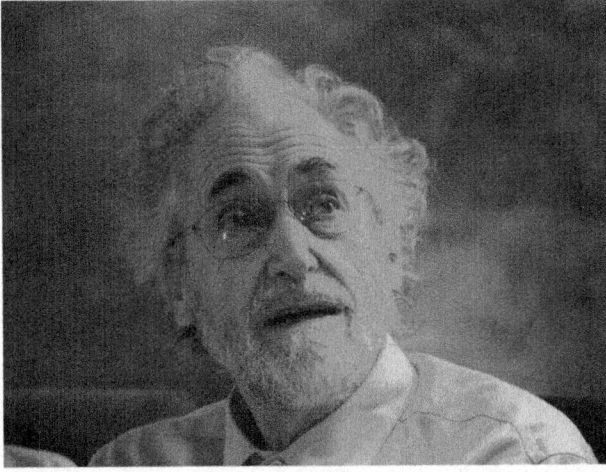

Dr Bob Johnson is a Consultant Psychiatrist and Visiting Professor at Bolton University where he was about to be made an Honorary Doctor of Science as this book went to press. A member of the Royal College of Psychiatrists and Royal College of General Practitioners he is also on the General Medical Council's Specialist Register for Psychiatry.[1] His qualifications include his degree from Cambridge University, an MA in Psychology, PhD in Medical Computing, and a Diploma in Psychotherapy, Neurology and Psychiatry from the Institute of New York. Details of his many articles, books and videos appear in *Appendix 1*.

'Dr Bob' is a former Head of Therapy, Ashworth Maximum Security Hospital and Consultant, Special Unit, Parkhurst Prison. The story of his ground-breaking work with dangerous offenders is told in (his wife) Sue Johnson's acclaimed *The Prison Psychiatrist's Wife* (Waterside Press, 2023).

---

1. Robert Alfred Johnson Registered No. 0400150.

Publisher's note

The views and opinions in this book are those of the author and not necessarily shared by the publisher. Readers should draw their own conclusions concerning the possibility of any competing accounts or explanations.

Acknowledgements

I would like to thank three special people without whom this book would not have appeared at this time. First my remarkable wife, Sue, whose penetrating account of our journey to Parkhurst Prison in 1991, *The Prison Psychiatrist's Wife* gives an all too graphic description of the needless destructions inherent in our myopic prison strategy. The book regularly brings a tear to my eye, since it gives free rein to cowardly bullies in high places. Happily it caught the eye of my publisher Bryan Gibson of Waterside Press who proved wonderful to work with, both in seeing the merit in Sue's book, and working hard to sort it editorially. His rubric, 'Putting justice into words', fits so closely with what I've been trying to do that it delights me. And finally, Leila Lee, then editor-in-chief of the academic journal *Philosophy Study*. Without Leila's consistent and reliable enthusiasm for my ideas, and the way I thought through problems, then this book would have been less than half as weighty. In all, she elicited ten such papers—three in 2020, five in 2021 and two in 2022. As with Bryan, I came to know that what I wrote would receive serious attention. This increased my confidence no end, such that it has enabled me to grow conclusions and coherences that would otherwise have eluded me.

I need also to acknowledge the UK's 1944 Education Act which was passed in the teeth of war. This brilliantly insightful statute funded my extraordinary education. As a hyper-idealistic youth, I was far too puritanical to even begin to contemplate incurring a huge mountain of student debt. I would probably have become a bricklayer. In today's topsy turvy world, we charge students fees for the price of working hard—myopic to the point of lunacy. So, my thanks to these three, to the politicians of 1944, and to the thousands of others who taught me all I know or refurbished what I thought anew.

Thanx

Dr Bob Johnson

June 2023

I dedicate this book to my wider planetary family, and wish them all well.

Foreword

Martin Brunt

I first saw Bob Johnson, many years ago, across the floor of an Old Bailey courtroom, a fitting place to meet a man who's immersed himself in the study of violence. Bob was a rare thing in that austere setting, the only person there trying to explain the reasons behind the brutality of the UK's most notorious prisoner Charles Bronson. Most of us were just along for the spectacle. Despite Bob's efforts, Bronson is still misunderstood by his jailers and banged up in maximum security, while the good doctor has gone on to develop his pioneering work on a bigger stage.

It was Leonardo Da Vinci who first said that 'everything connects to everything else'—his own genius for making remote but important connections being well-documented. In this innovative and highly informed account, 'Dr Bob'—as he's known to colleagues, patients and his many admirers—makes telling connections between warmongers, serial killers and other dangerous individuals. All suffer from the effects of 'Toddler Thinking', 'Nursery Nightmares' and 'Guff Disease'. This can be traced to their childhoods—*friendless childhoods explain warring adults*. Putin's war in Ukraine and Hitler's in Europe share the same origins as the violence done by 'monsters' in our deepest dungeons. Harm done to them at an early age persists into adulthood.

Bob authenticates this with excerpts from his conversations—'dialogues'—with some of the UK's most notorious serial killers. Work so unsettling for official thinking on crime and punishment that he found his unit at Parkhurst Prison summarily closed. Bob himself faced threats to invoke the Official Secrets Act for letting *Panorama* feature his professional records. For weeks he was front page news and there are many in the field that have never forgotten what was done to him, his colleagues, the prison system and penal policy. 'Tough on crime' began here.

So, violence Bob informs us, is born of childhood experiences that trigger adult anger, grievances and the destruction of the lives of others. He suggests how all killing — through war, or crime — can be avoided: by building truth, trust and consent for all. Ensuring we develop nutritious emotions not seeds of hate and aggression. To explore the darkest side of human nature he analyses excerpts from *Mein Kampf*, Shakespeare, George Orwell and his own professional notes. Prepare yourself to make connections and for a roller-coaster ride of facts, theories, findings and heartfelt explanations.

Hold on tight!

The author of the Foreword

Martin Brunt is crime correspondent for Sky News having been chief reporter at the *Sunday Mirror*. He has a longstanding reputation as an investigative journalist and being 'first on the scene'.

Preface

When Vladimir Vladimirovich Putin invaded Ukraine on Thursday 24 February 2022 people assumed that he, at least, knew why—commentators, however, were puzzled. What he said he was doing differed markedly from what was actually happening. And continues to do so, the more he talks. He lies—why? These events repeat, almost exactly, what happened in 1939—the invasion of a neighbouring country by Germany, for reasons that made no sense then or now. Have we learnt nothing since? Today, we have even less idea of where war comes from, and how it can realistically be stopped, than we did then. Time and technology don't help. At the present rate, we're blundering into thermonuclear annihilation, for all.

This book offers a healthier way through—it regards war and killing as a disease. It is based on my five years' work as a doctor in Parkhurst Prison UK asking 50 murderers why they killed. This required me to spend some 2,000 hours (including up to 700 hours which were video-recorded) discussing highly emotive topics—unaccompanied—with men who were serving life for murder. Few doctors have done this. By unpacking childhood traumas in this way, violence was eliminated from a maximum-security prison wing—no alarm bells were rung there for three years, down from 20 a year for the preceding seven—a success which could not have happened without explicit clarification of ferocious emotions.

Since 2020, I have published approaching 100,000 words in academic journals on and around this topic. This book is based on these earlier papers, which readers are free to peruse, should they wish. The conclusion offered here is both simple and stark—friendless childhoods explain warring adults. Violence and tyranny are seen as continuations into adult life of strategies and objectives learnt in desperate kindergartens. It is striking how often prominent politicians are depicted as infants—sometimes even in nappies (diapers). Most astonishing is how Hitler describes his appalling childhood, in his own words—*Mein*

Kampf was never more unexpected—I am grateful to Alice Miller for showing me this (see *Chapter 4*).

But this book comes with a serious medical warning. Flaunting nuclear warheads has dire medical consequences—medically speaking, radioactivity disintegrates the very proteins of which we, and our plants, are made, to say nothing of our DNA. To survive our very own lethal folly, we need to acknowledge, highlight and thereafter tackle, our prevalent Muddled Thinking, urgently.

The world in which we live is unduly *complex*. Too often, it afflicts us with Covid, Cancer, Climate Change, Crime, Corruption and Conflict—this book does not pretend otherwise. Instead, it seeks to identify the man-made elements in all of these, and by highlighting them—to ease them. The opening chapter shows the scope. The middle chapters might be heavy going. The last chapters revel in optimistic delight—if you find the first passages uphill, then you can always skip to the end, and tackle them later, as you wish.

Happy reading.

Dr Bob Johnson
June 2023

CHAPTER 1

Toddlers Squabble, Adults Socialise

---

*Inside The Suicide Bomber's Mind — Stumbling Toddlers — Nutritious
Emotions — How to Spot Toddler-thinking*

Inside The Suicide Bomber's Mind

'WE, THE SUPREME COURT OF THE UNITED STATES, insist that
killing people must be stopped — however, because we're Muddled Thinkers,
we've decided to have you killed, anyway.'

Now you might agree with this — but have a care, it is precisely the twisted
illogic that is an indispensable precondition for war. War cannot occur without
it. Remove it, and war goes and doesn't come back. However, unless we unpack
it, we're lost. Stalin killed Trotsky, Vladimir Putin kills Ukrainians — neither
could give you a good clear reason for doing so — because there isn't one.
Which is exactly what I found with the 50 murderers I worked with, for five
years, in Parkhurst Prison on the Isle of Wight. They too, didn't know why
they killed. Of course, they had plenty of 'answers', just as the US Supreme
Court does — but it's all guff. It doesn't add up. And if you regard killing people as a disease, which I do, then you need to know precisely where it's coming
from — i.e. a most accurate diagnosis — else the problem will end you as well.
This book describes what I winkled out from all those murderers — and if
something similar isn't applied globally, and soon, we're self-inflicted fossils.
Unclear thinking kills — whereas clarity cures.

Make no mistake about it — if you thought Hitler was horrific — imagine
him with a nuclear button. The world was already unsafe in 1939 — international treaties weren't worth the paper they were written on, progress was dire,
and calamity ensued. But nowadays, we face worse. Radioactive farmland is
a contradiction in terms — irradiated soil grows neither crops nor livestock,

only famine. Indeed, doctors use radiation to sterilise medical equipment. By unleashing nuclear weapons, leaders risk starving us all. Is that really a sensible human outcome? Can't we, as a species—a 'thinking' species at that—do better?

The point about Hitler, as later chapters explore, was that he didn't care. Or rather, he no longer cared. He did once, but that was fiercely buried in his past. It follows that appeals to his 'better nature', or what might pass as a conscience, are a waste of breath. They mattered when he was small, they mattered desperately—he says so in his own words. But that was long, long ago, and no longer applied when he waged war. And yet international relations are still conducted on the basis that irrational monsters are still thinking straight. We offer them a quid pro quo—you do this, and we'll do that. Or more usually, if you don't stop doing that, we'll punish you even more, or at least try to. The assumption is that they *are* thinking straight; that they *can* respond in a quasi-logical way, and thereupon discard the twisted illogic which launched them in the wrong direction, to begin with.

But this fractured thinking is different. It runs to a different tune. It's like a misguided missile—off-target in a fundamental way. Above all, it makes no sense—it's illogic. Hitler conceived a monster plan—he called it the Final Solution—but it didn't *solve* anything—how could it? Its sole purpose was to kill people—millions of them, systematically, on an expensive, industrial scale. Step back a minute and ask, 'What precise benefit did this extravagance bring to Hitler personally, let alone emotionally?' (i.e. — 'Why do it?') This is the key, because if we don't understand this, then we'd have no chance of offering either him, or his successors, a more effective remedy—one which might have some chance of deflecting them all.

Our normal assumption about human beings is that they like doing some things, and dislike others. You might call it motivation. And at its heart is staying alive. At least that's what we all commonly assume. Certainly, it's the basis of the medical profession, in which I have happily participated for many years.

Let's all agree that everyone of us values health. We put longevity at the top of our priorities—we save for our pensions, we bump up against our fellows, we grunt through our daily exercises, we watch our weight—all on the happy, idealistic assumption that we want to live longer. Doesn't everyone? Can we assume that however varied we humans are, or become, that at heart—when it comes down to it—we all prefer life to its alternative. But do we?

Bang into this idealism comes the suicide-bomber. She or he, by their very action, says suicide is my highest ideal. Longevity is for the birds—I'm for being killed today, rather than waiting (or working) for a better future. You might not agree with them—I certainly don't. I regard it as faulty reasoning, illogical. But there they are—recurring with sickening frequency. They are no longer using their ineffable human reasoning to enhance their own, or their victims' lives—but to end them. How can this be? Where does it come from?

And they pose a fundamental challenge to our thinking. How is it that though the vast majority of people do value life above killing, a persistent minority don't? Where does this discrepancy come from? Because if we can't uncover that, then the whole issue of nuclear weaponry will trundle on, in its terminal way, without any rational intervention on our part.

Of course, once the suicide-bomber has bombed, there's no way we can scrutinise their mind. It's a shut book. We can speculate. We can fume. We can grieve. But understanding is closed, at least for that episode. Again, the whiffs of 'reasonings' that do filter out, don't really add up. They are just as much guff as any other killer's 'reasons'. Differences in theology, differing expectations of life after death, or notions that civilisation can be improved by demolishing part of it—these appear to have convinced the bombers to kill themselves. Again, we normally expect weightier data, better arguments before we commit to such drastic action—so why is it lacking here? It is as absent here, as with all other examples of twisted illogic—and in this book, they all come from one, and only one, source.

Suppose you could catch a suicide bomber just before they bombed—what then? Well, I haven't managed to achieve this, any more than I have been able to interrogate Putin, Hitler or any number of other tyrants or demagogues. But what I have done, and this is the spine of this book, is to question in depth and at length, murderers—those who fully intended to kill, not necessarily themselves, though that follows often enough, but others of our fellows, *including on three occasions, myself.* Some, the serial killers, planned to do so repeatedly.

One man who I was fortunate enough to question in this way was especially illuminating. I call him Alec. Aged 24 he arrived in the Special Unit in Parkhurst Prison, after I had already been working there for some 18 months.

I was therefore able to video every interchange I had with him. And verbatim dialogue of his first and later sessions is revealing. I go into this in more detail in my book *How Verbal Physiotherapy Works.*

Alec says: '… but like I said, I said since I've been in prison, that, yes, I'll kill again, I know I'll kill again. And a part of me wants to kill again. And as long as that part wants to, *then I will let it.*'

Look carefully at these explicit words. All prospect of 'normal' restraints has gone. Alec contradicts our normal presumption of health — he doesn't see killing as unhealthy, it's something he does. He shows no interest in why 'a part of me wants to kill again' — he just accepts that this is how the world is, and, as long as it is that way — 'then I will let it'.

You could react in horror, you could close the whole thing down, as the then UK Government did my Parkhurst work, hoping it would all go away. Or, if you were interested in how healthy thinking disintegrates in this way, then you could explore where it all started. And, like everyone else, Alec had a childhood. And though children are often neglected, too often as a matter of the policies of Governments — here we put them and the foundation stones of their thinking, centre stage, since that, after all, is where we all began.

Stumbling Toddlers

ONCE YOU ADMIT THAT SOME HUMANS really don't mind killing other humans, once you concede that this does occur, however much we might wish it didn't — why then, if you're like me, you want to know why. You want to know where it comes from — because, if you don't know that, then you've no chance of stopping it. But murder raises the most powerful emotions there are — and ferocious emotions are the enemy of clarity — so it takes an effort of will, to hold your nose, and venture deeper into the horrors. Let's cut to the chase, and go straight into the nursery.

To find where illogical mayhem occurs on a regular, almost expected basis, all we need do is visit a badly run kindergarten. There, the bigger toddlers can always grab your favourite toy without difficulty — unless teacher stops them in time — you being too small to say no. Might is right. Toddlers squabble.

No-one can deny that. They do it all the time, at the drop of a hat — look the other way for a moment, and they're at it.

'That's mine.'
'No, it's not.'
'Give it me back.'
'Shan't.'
'Oh, for Goodness sake, why can't you lot behave.'
'Waaaaah.'

You might suppose that what happens routinely when we're all very small is a far cry from mobilising armies, and loosing off missiles — but we were all toddlers once, when putting one foot in front of the other took our full concentration. Even then we wobbled. Now both security and defence are more controversial, and more emotionally fraught than anything else — so if we can find things we *can* all agree on, then we need to put them centre stage, give them top priority, if we are to have any chance of getting through. And if recalling when you were a toddler eludes you, there are plenty of living examples around, to feast your eye on — all freely available, and carrying within them a dark but otherwise obvious secret.

And wherever you come from, whatever your philosophy or politics, you cannot deny that we all start off very small. At birth, we are none of us much above 60 cms (two feet) tall, if that. Of course, we progress, we grow, we get bigger. We learn to walk across the room without having to collapse on to all fours, and crawl about, like we did at first. But none of us are born bipedal — we have to learn. And moving from the one to the other is not straightforward. It's easy to forget just how difficult it was — indeed, there is a huge incentive to do so. Aged two, or younger, you see all the other toddlers moving around like these unbelievable adults do — as if there was nothing to it — so you are on your mettle to do the same.

But it's hazardous. That ground can be very hard. Grazed knees are your constant companion. That foot takes some controlling — it doesn't always go where you want it to, and you collapse. Very un-dignifying. Not to be dwelt on, nor talked about. Keep it dark. Whoops — there's the key to *muddled thinking*.

Watch how that slipped in. Something that is obvious to everyone else, a trick that is nothing to be ashamed of, suddenly becomes something you don't like to think about. You feel vulnerable. You see yourself at a disadvantage. Others sail across the room, without a problem—they have a bipedal confidence which you dearly wish you had—but there you go again, tumbling, stumbling and falling about.

Don't minimise that chagrin, the mental pain—nor how you can so easily try and make it go away. Just don't think it through—that'll get rid of it, that'll move it out from mocking you. It gets lost, it no longer features, it's gone. But has it? It may have gone from your very own mental world, but the reality with which we all have to cope is something else. It carries on, as it does, whether we like it or not—and the real solution is not to pretend, to wishful-think, to lie to oneself, but to open your eyes to what's really happening, what's really going on—because that's the final arbiter. Not what you wish, or what I would pontificate on—but what's real.

The central theme of this book is that unclear thinking bedevils us. But there's no point in only depicting what goes wrong—we can all see that all too clearly—the question is—why? And having established why, let's look at the cure. That's standard medical practice—find out the nature of the disease, otherwise known as the diagnosis, and then, based on the accuracy of this assessment, intervene to ameliorate.

Later in the book, we look at some really gruesome scenarios—unhappily the world seems to have too many of them—scenes where A does unspeakable things to B, and doesn't seem to turn a hair. What is going on? Well that's what the book sets out to explore. So at these foot hills, let's keep it nice and simple, so that we all know what's going on, and can see for ourselves what's needed, and what isn't.

Let's stick with toddlers to start with. We can see their struggles, where we can't remember our own. When robots were first being invented, getting them to walk on two legs was found to be surprisingly difficult. It is. It requires accurate coordination of virtually all the muscles in your body, and then an ability to throw yourself forwards, in the full anticipation you will land securely. There's no guarantee you will. But that's what's required.

And then, one glorious day, one you may well have long forgotten—you walk. You glide from room-to-room, or across the fields, without a care in the world. Toddling becomes a thing of the past. No longer are you struggling to travel — two legs are so much more efficient for locomotion. Freeing up your arms and hands is a wonderful improvement — you can suddenly use them for grabbing things, for feeding yourself and for other wondrous activities — activities which are simply unavailable if you need them to support half your weight for moving yourself about.

But look at what it takes. Standing on your own two feet — listen to the emotions which such a well-worn phrase carries. Being responsible for your own travel — once you can walk, you can place yourself where you want, not where others put you. It's easy to forget what a difference this makes. But, not only is the change dramatic — so is the chasm that persists, if you can't make it. What would happen if you never really made it onto two legs, but were destined to spend the rest of your life scrabbling around on all fours? Think about it. What a humiliation. What a come down. What a tragedy. What if your emotions were still going on all fours? What if you were approaching the rest of your life, as if you were still, emotionally, only two feet (60 cms) tall? It happens.

And that's where wars come from.

Nutritious Emotions

SO FAR, NOTHING MYSTERIOUS, nothing spectacular, nothing that you or I haven't seen a million times. Toddlers have difficulty walking about. What could be peculiar about that? They are also invariably much shorter than the people looking after them — who can deny that? If toddlers aren't fed, watered and looked after, they do not survive. Yes, we're talking survival. And just as the emotions which accompany murder are huge, those that attend staying alive are equally overwhelming. In fact, that's what emotions are for — to warn you, to press you to further effort, to galvanise you out of your rut into a safer zone. Or what they think is a safer zone. But how do they know? Well, like we know everything else — it's what we've found to be the case in the past. We assume it'll be similar if not identical. And that's life saving, when it's real — and deadly when it's not. If you're not frightened of walking across a busy main road, you're not long for this world.

This is where the problem gets stuck — why do some of us fail to catch up emotionally? We all start small, yes. We also grow — some more healthily than others. And in doing so, our emotional world matches our physical world — the two are in tandem, certainly to begin with. In fact, you might even go so far as to say that when we are first born, all we have to speak of are emotions. We smile, we wail, we 'Waaaaah' — without the least difficulty. Again, nothing unexpected about that. Indeed, in the old days, midwives used to smack newborns to make sure they cried — not exactly the best welcome into our difficult world, but there.

Not only do we channel emotions as our primary means of communication — we also sense them with a precision that verges on the uncanny. We may not have language, as in words and sentences — but we listen to the emotions behind what is said — either to us, at us, or at anyone else in the room. In fact, I can't help noting that, even in the womb, we hear the voices of our parents, or those near enough to our very own mother's abdominal wall — yes, we every one of us did have one of those, a long time ago. Medically speaking we grow our ears some eight weeks after conception, and you may be sure we use them for the next 32 weeks, with ever-increasing assiduity.

Emotions exist and are fully operational at birth. At that time, they are invariably at a maximum. They are always sizeable when other people are in charge of our survival. How could it not be? Are we going to be fed? Are we going to be given a comfortable bed for the night? Does this matter? I should say it does — to begin with it matters 100%. You may be able to 'Waaaaah' when you first arrive — but you sure as heck can't feed yourself. Indeed, human infancy is a prolonged transfer of responsibility from adult carers, usually parents, to yourself. When this transition goes smoothly and well, then your emotions grow along with your body — you learn how to feed yourself both calory-wise, and emotionally.

But what if the transfer is faulty? What then? Ah ha — that's the key. Hitler describes in gruesome detail how he was mis-educated emotionally — and if it didn't work for him, why is it a surprise that it doesn't work for such as Alec, or indeed Putin and his ilk. Transfer — that's what you need. And what you find, at least what I found, was that faulty transition from toddler to adult, accounts for *muddled thinking*, what you might more properly call Toddler-Thinking.

This is such an important juncture in human development, that you would expect to find buckets of evidence to illuminate it—emotional support in infancy influencing later life. But the way we've been moving in thinking about these potent matters, hasn't helped. The shock of the First World War drove philosophers to a very narrow view of humanity—first define your terms, else you're talking nonsense. Sounds sensible, but it comes to grief when you talk emotion. Emotions have more shapes than a pint (or litre) of water, so if you insist on defining them before even discussing them, then you're sunk—and so are the people you are trying to help, let alone understand. You'd be surprised how many suffer from this 'scientific' emotional blindspot.

So let's assume emotions exist, and are important. Where's the scientific evidence? Well, as you might expect, there's a colossal amount—but you have to look in the right direction, else you'll miss it. Why not compare the different growth rates in children who are well fed with those who are half-starved? When you do this, it's obvious—restricting food intake hampers physical growth, as you'd fully expect. But here's the thing. Even when you replace the calories but neglect the emotions physical growth *does not* resume. Yes, you read that right. Emotions influence physical growth. It's called 'failure to thrive', psychosocial dwarfism, or, for the really technically minded—hypopituitarism (Johnson, 2022a).

Mark this well—if the emotional deficit, along with the food intake, is replenished, then physical growth is started again. You add inches or centimetres by prescribing *nutritious emotions*. Without these, growth is not increased by calories alone.

Well, how woolly can you get? Am I really suggesting that smiling at children helps them grow bigger? Really? If that were the case, you would find quantities of evidence that scowling at them kept them short. How could this be? Everyone knows that physical height requires nutritious food—where's the evidence that emotional input is just as important? Or, from the point of view of this book, even more so.

So let's take a large population of children—in the millions. Let's starve them for a few years. Then, when you start feeding them again, you divide them into two groups—the one has emotional support, the other emotional deprivation. Sounds heartless, which it is—but it has already been done. The whole population of German children was indeed deliberately starved during the First World War. Starvation was regarded as an acceptable wartime strategy, as it was during and after the Iraq War. In the 1920s, when feeding programmes were introduced, the evidence was overwhelming — at least it was for those prepared to listen. Growth resumed at an astonishing rate — adding several inches (or centimetres) to height, in a matter of months. Except — and note this most carefully — not in those whose emotions were restricted. Even the right calorie input didn't help. Physical evidence that emotions matter. They matter for physical size — how tall are you? They matter for emotional weight — how much do you matter?

Now it can't be over-emphasised that these are complex and highly emotional areas. Even the significance of emotions in themselves can struggle in some psychiatric quarters. So when they are put centre stage, as they are in this book, it is quite essential to move along very carefully, making sure that the points made follow logically one after another. Leaps into 'faith' based notions, or supposed outcomes, can soon end in muddle and confusion — so care must be taken as we go along to maintain contact, to keep the chain of reasoning intact, at least as far as possible.

To recap — *muddled thinking* bedevils adult behaviour. Next, emotional input in infancy is as important as food. Physical growth cannot occur if starved — *but* without *nutritious emotions*, all growth *will remain stunted*. Once the vital role of *nutritious emotions* has been established, then we can begin to look for pointers which show that reasoning too has got stuck — whence *toddler-thinking*, to which we now turn.

How to Spot Toddler-Thinking

TODDLING IS SIMPLE, but not easy. At one level, all you have to do is lift one foot off the floor, wave it in the air for a while, and then plonk it down again, hopefully a sensible distance in front of you so that you progress forwards, instead of sideways or even backwards. But this simplicity hides multiple complications. Lifting your feet up, even only one, means balancing precariously on another — thereby automatically increasing the chances of coming a cropper — whence all those grazed knees.

More, you have to have some idea of where to go, else this hazardous procedure offers much risk for little gain. And just look more closely at that risk. In order to walk, you have to leave the relative stability of a two-legged stance, where your weight is secured on two stalwart feet, to one in which you are actually falling. Yes, falling forwards. You have to leave the status quo with which you are by now largely familiar, for something new, something that hasn't been tried before. And in order to move yourself, your whole weight has to tip forwards, initially into thin air. Only with skill, do you then bring your leading foot forward soon enough to land securely, thereby breaking your fall, not your leg.

Complex, I should say so. Yet we all do it. We start crawling, and then we walk. Some of us even run marathons. But don't forget the initial stage, the first steps. They may sound ever so simple — but you only have to watch a toddler or two, to see that they can be anything but easy.

So what would help, and what hinder? Here is where *nutritious emotions* come to the fore. Place yourself back in the toddler position. You are desperate to succeed. But you soon learn that moving forwards can be painful. Gentle emotional encouragement can make all the difference. 'Come on, you can do it' — and other such cheerful phrases can make a material difference. Compare these with scorn, with sneers — 'Oh, you're hopeless, you'll never learn to walk' — mockery can so easily warp you for life — which is where all the trouble begins.

So if *nutritious emotions* have such importance, not only in toddling successfully, but also in growing to the full height that our genes permit — what are they? Where's the scientific definition that will make all scientists, psychologists, psychiatrists, philosophers and indeed everyone you can think of — sit up, and say, 'Yes, *nutritious emotions* are what we all need, throughout life, but especially in infancy when we're learning how to cope with the knocks and setbacks which are inherent in our Uncertain Universe.'

If you follow the modern tradition, you tend to insist on first defining your terms. If *nutritious emotions* are so vital for health, what do they consist of, where do they come from, and how can you spread them around? A similar scepticism attended penicillin in the early days — no-one had ever heard of a drug which only attacked infections, leaving the human entirely unscathed. It sounded too good to be true — a drug which helped but didn't cause harm. It sounded like any other wishful-thinking—would you invest serious resources in it, just because it sounded good?

As before, since powerful emotions can bedevil calm considerations, we need if possible to cool the discussion down to the simplest level possible, and take matters from there, ensuring, wherever we can, that the thread continues intact. So let's start with what everyone knows—food. How would you define what food is? Well, keeping matters simple, it's what you put in your mouth. Because if you don't, you starve. Seems quite elementary. You eat, because if you don't, you are first ill, then dead. Brutal, but medically indisputable.

Now food is solid, obvious and every day. You can see it, weigh it, chew it. Emotions seem so insubstantial by comparison—but check them out. Next time you are fed emotions you find to be indigestible, just see how long you chew them over—it can be years. So don't make the mistake that too many 'professionals' do—that because you cannot measure them, they don't impact. Emotions matter. In fact they are what make the difference between what's of value, and what isn't. Indeed, even the word itself gives the game away—*emotion*—it's what *moves* you.

If *nutritious emotions* are what you need to navigate toddling successfully, or more precisely, healthily—then it should be no surprise to find they continue to play a similar role with all the other challenges that this curious life throws into our path, for the rest of our life. And here we link the thread with the question of killing. Look again at what Alec says earlier in this chapter about being moved to kill. As long as that part of him is there, he will let it move him to kill. How about introducing an emotion, a 'moving', which stopped that part of him wanting to kill?—that'd be a saving.

What stops Alec and so many others from catching up? Why do negative emotions linger so long? If they inflict so much *muddled thinking*, surely their owner would spot this, and reprise. All it would take is synchronising with adult reality, where what you did, or didn't do, was no longer curtailed by what your parents or carers thought or decided—it'd be up to you. In emotional terms, you would be standing on your own two feet. Splendid idea, excellent pathway to health.

But that's just what *toddler-thinkers* don't do. They get stuck. Like Alec, they see the world in one way, and as long as that's there, they let it dictate what they do, what they see, and indeed what they say. The answer to this was not easy to find—it took me three decades of searching. The practical fact is, that there is something serious which stops them—something too deep to dig up casually. It's too painful to think about—so you don't. You keep going the way you've always done—keep the parent-figments sweet, and you may live to see the next day. But get caught out, and parental-type wrath, *disapproval*, will finish you. This is a vaguely 'seen' hazard, an ill-thought-through threat that happens to have been true, for all the time you were a toddler. It just happens also to be false once you're an adult. But it's that transition which makes the difference—and one you cannot achieve without *nutritious emotions*. As an infant, you can safely go about on all fours—toddling is risky. The same applies to emotions—what you know, what you've been taught by the most important people in your life at that critical time, predominates, until you can stand on your own two feet, and thereafter question and so revise it. Clarity cures, but is hard to come by.

Note too, that talking fast and loose can get you off the hook. And this is where lies come from. Those who are emotionally adult know that this is a complicated world. It needs reliable and *truthful* checking, to make sure that what you're doing is working, is making a difference and is helping. *Reality* matters most. This is entirely opposite to what happens in the toddler's world. For toddlers, the number one priority is keeping the 'authorities' sweet—mum and/or dad comprise your entire universe—get them wrong, and you're toast. *Approval* matters most.

Alec's words (reproduced earlier) then become, 'A part of me wants to *lie*. And as long as that part wants to, *then I will let it.*' Lying doesn't relate to this world, it comes from an imaginary world, where you can pretend that *nutritious emotions* are abundant—sadly, the desperate toddler has to make-believe such a world, because the reality they then see, is otherwise. Hitler describes why, to a tee. The real Catch 22 is that in order to dispense with *toddler-thinking*, you need to have oodles of *non-toddler-thinking*—which is precisely what you haven't got. What you need most is harsh reality—*the truth* of the matter. What you've got, generally, is toddler-truths—truths which were perfectly true when you were a toddler—mum and/or dad were your world—but now you need to stand on your own two feet—but who can tell you this? Who would you listen to? Who would you TRUST? You know how easy it is to lie—doesn't everybody?

This chapter has explored the foothills. The next one asks how *nutritious emotions* apply to war. As the climbing gets steeper, the exploration expands to examine why the impact of revenge is so powerful, and why *consent*, and above all *clarity*, are more so. The maxim running throughout this book on killing, is the one that Covid should have taught us all—i.e. that no-one-is-safe-until-we're-all-safe. Finally, for the more intrepid reader who does reach the summit, the perspective from there is intended to justify the climb, since it unpacks that redolent phrase—no-one-is-sane-until-we're-all-sane.

CHAPTER 2

Don't Drop Bombs — Drop White Goods

Why Did Alec Want to Garrotte Me? — Digestible Emotions — War,
An Expensive Way of Making Things Worse — 'When I Meet
Someone Without a Smile, I Give Them One Of Mine'

Why Did Alec Want to Garrotte Me?

WHAT WOULD YOU DO if a serial killer, such as Alec, made meticulous plans to kill you? Would you:

(a) Shoot him/her?
(b) Scarper?
(c) Seek help?

When you're under attack, it's not easy to think things through — priorities take over, and they push you into immediate and urgent action. It's what those life-saving emotions are for. One pull of the trigger, and it's all over for you. However, in this book, we can take our time, turn things over more carefully, look at the wider picture and consider the optimum. As a doctor, you see many horrendous things — indeed you start off your career in the dissecting room, coping with a whole series of dead bodies — at least I did. Then in the operating theatre, you might witness, as I did as a medical student, the steady demise of a previously healthy woman. Bad things do happen. People do die. And people do kill people. The question is, what do you do about it? Not what your immediate, emotional, even panic reaction is — but what would a sane, sensible person do? What is really going on? What is actually at stake? And what's the way through — if there is one?

Well, if you regard killing people, for whatever reason, as a disease, then medical reasoning takes over. All disease is unhealthy, by definition. All diseases have causes, usually several, and it's your job, as a doctor, to sort them into a practical order, tackle the immediate ones first, and then secure the best treatment available. It doesn't always work, but that shouldn't discourage you — because, more often than not, it does, and each success adds to your confidence, your delight, and your willingness to press onwards.

When Alec began practicing garrotting his pillow, preparatory to silencing me, I didn't hesitate. It was not my job to shoot him, nor to run away — so I sought help — which, happily for us both, was immediate, and, crucially, trustworthy. It happened like this. For about a year, Alec had been coming to my office on the prison wing, faithfully every week. We inched around his determination to kill every two years by taking tentative steps into his hideous childhood. Nothing too drastic, just a willingness to listen. Gentle probing to show I had total confidence that there was something going on underneath, which Alec needed to see, but, so far, could not.

Unhappily for me, I had gone too fast. I didn't know I had. It's just that Alec abruptly stopped coming to see me. In a coercive environment such as a maximum-security prison wing, there is precious little room for consent, which I regarded as indispensable. Because of this I devised a system of appointments for prisoners to come to see me. They only had to walk down the wing and knock on the door to my 'office', which was actually just another cell, like the one they were passing their life sentences in. And being a wing of a maximum-security prison, there was nowhere else for them to go, nor anything else for them to do. But offering them an appointment did give them a say in what happened, at least in that aspect of their life. So, when Alec declined for a month, I knew something was amiss. And it was.

Rumours spread through the wing that Alec was going to agree to come and start seeing me again. But, as I turned to switch my beloved video camera on, he would garrotte me from behind. Now I knew he planned everything, meticulously. His earlier murder in prison had been carefully scheduled — he knew where the hammer was kept, when the man would be most vulnerable, and how hard he had to keep hitting him. In fact, if you've the stomach for it, he had told me earlier that he planned to kill every two years — that was his aim in life, and, as he put it, as long as 'it' wanted to, he would let it. 'As you are falling asleep,' he said, 'you might be planning your next holiday. When I am, I plan my next murder.'

He was quite clear how things would work out. He would kill in one prison, and then be moved to the next. There, some unfortunate would say the wrong thing, mispronounce his name, fail to say good morning when he should have done—and bingo, that would trigger the procedure—meticulous planning—which he seemed to enjoy as much as the killing. And when he started putting me in the crosshairs, I took him very, very seriously. It wasn't that I hadn't said good morning 'correctly'—what I had done was ask the wrong questions about his mother—or perhaps they were the right ones, though not *necessarily* in the right order.

I have to admit that this episode called for expertise rather outside my normal medical skills, so I sought help. Now prisons are just like other large, rigid institutions—you get some good apples and some less so. As luck would have it, the man currently in charge of the entire prison was not the normal Governor, but the deputy—a man who had a flair for innovation. His April fool jokes were legendary. Thus, when I told him I no longer felt comfortable walking down the wing to get myself a cup of tea he assured me he would take care of the problem in the middle of the following week. This riled me, as he had anticipated it would. I don't usually get worked up, but I did. *Not next week*, I remonstrated, *now!* He had been joking. He moved swiftly into effective action. He ordered Alec into the segregation block that night, told him I would visit in the morning, and report back to him. And he would then decide what to do with Alec. Remarkable man.

The following day I was tidying papers in my office when three prisoners knocked on my door in close succession. 'I see myself as Alec, 30 years ago,' said one, 'If he goes through the rest of his life sentence, having threatened to kill the doctor, his life will be hell.' They none of them pressured me. They sought to persuade. In essence, they looked for my consent—in a coercive jungle, this was a rare jewel. Just like a village. 'He needs to come back to this Special Unit.'

As instructed by the deputy governor, I duly went round to the 'block', armed myself with two robust staff members, and gingerly opened Alec's cell door. The thing to guard against is a prisoner rushing out, as soon as they hear the door being unlocked, and attacking the newcomers before they can react. We stood well back. Nothing like this occurred. There was Alec, sitting crestfallen

33

on the bed and I went and sat next to him. 'I shouldn't have done that,' he said, 'I've done two years in solitary before—but I can't take it anymore. I need to get back to the unit.'

I told him, in formal tones, that I would inform the deputy governor, and he would decide what to do next. If you have any notion of the bureaucratic mayhem that prisons labour under, you need to treble it with regards to this Special Unit. Happily, however we were in safe hands, and the deputy governor took it upon himself to breach all protocols. And having transferred Alec out, promptly transferred him back in, to continue our journey together, on which more anon.

Digestible Emotions

LET'S BE CLEAR—I DIDN'T STOP Alec garrotting me by showering him with smiles or soft talk. No, I had him forcibly removed from the scene, using muscle and coercive authority that I did not myself possess, nor did I aspire to. I had no compunction in this. I was doing what any ordinary toddler would do, if you swiped their favourite toy—I'd appeal to the adult-in-the-room, the teacher. And in fact, naughty boys (and girls) do need a 'naughty corner' from time-to-time. But it must be commensurate and seen as fair by the recipient. Alec knew all about solitary confinement—he'd been there many times before, so it was well within his expectations. Anything more by way of 'punishment' or 'retribution' would have damaged his nascent growth points beyond repair. And that's where our handling of aberrant, dangerous, or lethal behaviour goes wrong—we overreact, hammer the culprit into the ground, and then wonder why he, or she, doesn't grow, doesn't improve.

So *nutritious emotions* have to be *digestible*. Any 'naughty corner' has to be appropriate, fair, and within reasonable bounds, as expected by the culprit—otherwise you are merely reinforcing their dismal, toddler-view of this difficult world. I didn't want Alec to continue to believe that the world was arbitrarily against him, that nothing he could do would improve matters. But I did want him to learn that certain destructive behaviours were unacceptable, that they came from his toddler-past, and were not only out of date today, but they cemented him into his nursery nightmare. Precisely the same applies to war.

Suppose I had had overweening confidence in my medical skill, had 'known' why Alec wanted to kill me, and so set out to explain to him why his behaviour wasn't logical. What if I'd sat him down and tried to remonstrate with him. 'Look Alec,' I might have said, 'be reasonable. I'm only a doctor here, I'm just trying to help you. Can't we let bygones be bygones and start afresh? Let me appeal to your better nature, your common sense, your common decency. Any normal person would acknowledge my good intentions, and so try and keep me alive, instead of carefully plotting my demise. So why can't you?'

How would you rate my chances? Again, it's comforting to think that inside every human being, without exception, there is a gentle peace-loving individual trying to get out. But there is far too much evidence to the contrary. Far too much squabbling going on all the time. So that it's hard to even suggest there might be a healthier way through — though that is exactly what this book does. Wish me luck.

Let's go right back to the beginning and start afresh. What do all humans do? All the time? Without exception? There is a wide range of answers to this. Some you will agree with, and some I won't. Let's look at the most basic. Every human I've ever known breathes in and out. When they don't, they're either ill, or dead. There are a number of other 'vital' functions, which we all do, generally without thinking, which keep us alive. And when they don't, we label them diseased. I call this the health-view-of-morality. And as mentioned in the previous chapter, most people would agree. It's the ones that disagree — the people like Alec who kill (or lie) as easily as breathing — they are the ones who need sorting. If we don't have a better method of coping with them, then we're all toast.

Instead of bemoaning the sins of the world, let's look more closely at those who don't agree with this 'health' view of morals. Why do a minority think it's perfectly reasonable to kill, to go to war, or, as a prerequisite to both, to *muddle-think*?

Twisted illogic — that's where we go wrong. Alec, and others, killed or kill, because that's what part of them wanted to do. Similarly — too many people lie, and deceive — again because part of them wants to. So where does that destructive, illogical part come from? In this book, it comes not from genes nor from an alien nature, but exclusively from what they've learnt as toddlers, what they've been taught — either deliberately by equally misinformed parents, or inadvertently because their carers didn't know any better. And the remedy, indeed the cure offered here, goes by the name of 'Nutritious Emotions'.

What is obvious to all is that if you don't feed infants enough food, then they don't grow. What needs equal emphasis is the verifiable fact that if you deprive them of *nutritious motions*, they remain stunted. Calorie input has to be adequate — but on its own it's not sufficient. It's easy to be clear about proteins and other food-values — we can measure these, count them, weigh them to our heart's content — so there's no disputing the need for them when we're very small.

The trouble with emotions is that they are fluid, they swish to and fro, without too much rhyme or reason — and one person's definition, even description of one emotion, can differ radically, even violently, from another's. But this indefinability does not mean they don't matter. They matter enormously. In fact, they are vital. So much so that, just as physical bodies don't grow without sufficient calorie input — without adequate *nutritious emotions*, minds don't either.

The point needs hammering home. Too many people, scientists and others, hide behind the elusive nature of emotions — saying they are unscientific, or far too subjective. Besides there's so much negativity, so much active enmity around, that to base a whole medical approach on benignity is questioned. Well, I take comfort from the view, that this negating view has also been learned or taught — it's not intrinsic in human nature. I saw definitive evidence on this in Parkhurst — indeed, explicitly in Alec, and others.

More, precisely the same indefinability applies to everything else. You and I breathe oxygen in and carbon dioxide out, with very little, if any understanding of what these two important gasses are about. We don't even know their detailed subatomic structure — indeed no-one does, but that's a different story, and it's quite irrelevant to whether we are breathing enough to stay alive. We know when there's not enough oxygen — and we move to correct it. We react. Unless we're already dead. Precisely the same reasoning applies to *nutritious emotions* — I'm happy to attempt to *describe* them — but I don't care to *define* them — indeed I neither want to, nor am capable of defining them — but I know what I like, just as you do. And as with oxygen, I am well-aware when I am not getting enough. As, I venture to suggest, are you. All I've done is extend this reasoning to the time frame when we are all most vulnerable — when we're toddlers.

Next — having developed this optimistic view of the most dangerous prisoners in the entire UK prison system — how did I deliver it? And, in parallel, how should I set about convincing the sceptical reader of its relevance? Well, I developed a three-pronged approach, which I term 'Truth, Trust and Consent'. Is it *true* that *nutritious emotions* are essential for peace-of-mind? Are they crucial to mind-growth? Does their lack show up, decades later? My answer to all these is — Yes.

That's fine for me. But do you, gentle reader, *trust* my assertion? Well, trust is another curious item which you cannot buy, you can only earn. And it's not easy. You have to be consistent in the small things, you have to be reliable in everything you come into contact with — not easy, especially as we are all fallible human beings. And last but a long way from least, is *consent*. The other party has to consent to trust the truth of what you assert. Quite a narrow input channel. In a coercive, punitive, controlling environment, a big challenge. But again, the bigger the challenge, the greater the success, if you succeed.

So how would *nutritious emotions* apply internationally, if they are to have any prospect of increasing peace and reducing war? Well again, the need for truthfulness is overriding, else the recipients will not trust your best endeavours, nor therefore consent to forego bellicosity. And who can blame them?

But, if *nutritious emotions* could once be established to be of equal, if not greater, importance than physical nourishment, then human ingenuity could be deployed to deliver. My strategy would be to drop *white goods*, by which I mean cookers, washing machines, solar desalinators and other consumer wonders which make life so much less of a drudge. The point being that you wish to show your international neighbours that you come in peace, not war. That you want to improve life for them, not bomb them into the stone age. Only by doing so have you even half a chance of securing their consent, their consent not to attack you, but to respect what we should all have learnt from Covid — that no-one-is-safe-until-we're-all-safe.

Trustworthy consent — powerful stuff, if you can earn it — arguably the most powerful thing in our cosmos.

War — An Expensive Way of Making Things Worse

MONEY IS A RICH SOURCE OF MUDDLED THINKING. And it is easy to see why, once the basic parameters are thoroughly clarified. Money is essentially a substitute, a replacement. And it works very well, generally. I don't have to bake my own bread, nor grow all my own crops — I can earn money elsewhere and buy them. What a saving. What a wonderful mechanism for cooperating. We're a social species — we have neither fangs to defend ourselves, nor wings to fly us out of trouble. No, we have each other — separately we are vulnerable — cooperating socially, we can survive. This is the underlying medical truth behind the maxim — no-one-is safe-until-we're-all-safe. And money, especially sourced from many, and invested long-term, can improve both our chances, and also the quality, of our joint survival, out of all recognition.

Then, *bang*, into this simplistic and comforting scenario comes *nutritious emotions* — something you can never buy. Why not? Well, try the following. Will you smile at me, if I give you a million? Well, the simple answer is 'Of course'. But what have I just bought? Are you smiling at me because of me — or because of my money, which I now no longer have — having just given it away. Money can buy most things — but it cannot buy consent, nor trust, nor indeed truth. They all three have to be earned the hard way — and for that, you have to have the most *un-muddled-thinking* you can get.

Money of course, is highly emotive — and, as always, when emotions run high clarity suffers. Let's put money aside for a moment, and go back to basics, points we can all agree on, and which can serve as a clear, reliable and logical way forwards. The base truth on which this book relies is health — it is robustly assumed that we all prefer being well to being ill, to living rather than the reverse. We need to sort out why some of us go to war, but meanwhile let's agree that being healthy is something we all aspire to, something we will all work towards and enthusiastically support. A common universal goal for an often-squabbling species.

At our most basic, we are all mammals. We don't give birth to offspring who can run around and peck for their food like chickens. No, we have a long and often tortuous childhood, in which, crucially for this point, we need a free lunch. Yet a 'free lunch' is precisely what many throw around as a term of abuse, when arguing vociferously about how to spend, or not spend, our taxes.

How do you explain that? We none of us would have survived infancy with-out being fed for free, especially mother's milk — that's what being a mammal means. Breasts too are highly emotive, but in medical terms they are mammary glands, which nourish neonates better than any substitute. And, to be even blunter, that's all we can do, when we first arrive — suckle. We have no teeth, we have zero control of our limbs or other muscles — happily our tongues can suck, else we're dead.

Is that all we need? When first born, and forever after, are we only concerned to fill our stomachs, as our number one priority? Our overriding motivation? Some would tell you so and seek to make a lot of money in the process. Here, we differ — we immediately add emotions. Food is vital, but *nutritious emotions* even more so. At least they are from a health point of view. It is worth repeat-ing that children fed food, but not *nutritious emotions*, do not thrive. They may survive, but thriving, enjoying life, taking delight in our fellow creatures — that requires an adequate supply of elusive, indefinable, heart-warming emotions.

Again, all these theorised, comforting assertions call for concrete evidence. Let's then take a closer look at a newborn, someone who has just emerged into the harsh light of day, having been cosseted for nine months in his mother's womb. Meet Ethan. A stunning video shows how, within the first few seconds of life in the outside world, Ethan is squawking. He doesn't know what's going on, what's happening, or what to expect next. He is then put in his mother's arms. Miraculously, he promptly settles. He stops all his 'Waaaaah'. Wonderful. And then he confirms the central point of this book, as follows. His mother offers him her breast — but, as the commentary makes most clear, Ethan is much more interested in looking at his mother's face.

What? Has Ethan already got a mind? Is he already working things out? He's barely *five minutes old*, and he prefers to look at his mother rather than drink her milk. What a turnaround. What a different perspective on human beings. If you look closely at how we begin, then that will show you clearly enough, without room for dispute, that what goes on in our mind is more important that what goes into our mouths. Again, it's ethereal, it's intangible, it's eas-ily overlooked — but Ethan wants to know what's going on, even before he takes his very first meal. I love this video and show it at every opportunity I have—my thanks to Ethan and all, especially SocialBaby.com, which recorded it, and made it so freely available.[1]

And what does Ethan do next? He responds socially to his dad *within 17 minutes of being born*. When his father sticks out his tongue at his new son, Ethan reciprocates—he does exactly the same in response. He sticks out his own tongue—and for the sceptics among you, and to convince you that there's been no mistake—he repeats the same, a few minutes later. Ethan is making social contact. He is relating to his fellow humans. If this doesn't bring a tingle down your spine, perhaps it should. The only muscle he can reliably control, else he couldn't suckle, is his tongue. And here he is using it to 'answer' an invitation from his dad to relate, to converse, to socialise. Being social matters immediately we are born. What a tragedy that so many of us forget—we needn't, indeed if we want to survive as a species, we'd far better not.

Money often goes right—but here it goes wrong. Too many accumulate cash so as to buy what we never had—compensate with cash for comforts—wrong department—comfort food is just food—comfort, and indeed peace-of-mind comes from the *triple values—truth, trust and consent*. You can earn them, but only when you put them centre stage. Not when you're still preoccupied with 'buying' them. Or convincing yourself that they're not really that important anyway, you've never had them before—so why start now? Well, for one thing delight needs to be taught, and needs *nutritious emotions* to flourish—and that makes it fun in itself. And next, if you delight in other human beings, which happen to be the only, or at least the essential source of *nutritious emotions*, then you won't want to kill them off, bomb them, or otherwise delete them as possible sources of what everyone of us must have to keep a stable mind. Here is the start of the second maxim—no-one-is-sane-until-we're-all-sane.

With these basic human facts in mind, money can be seen in a different light, so can the costs of war. Money has no intrinsic value—you can't eat gold. We assign money to a whole variety of symbols, from seashells to binary digits—it has zero value in itself, except where we humans allow. Which leads on to say that in all transactions—commercial, social, belligerent—the vital factor is what other living humans do. They are the only ones who can possibly deliver

---

1. Robson L (2013), Social baby, YouTube: https://www.youtube.com/watch?v=RtwXnTUojFo The original of this 'second generation' video is included in Murray L and Andrews L, *The Social Baby: Understanding Babies' Communication from Birth*: see https://www.socialbaby.com/the-social-baby-interactive.html

nutritious emotions. And, though too many don't know what *nutritious emotions* are, or dismiss them as something they've never met, and keep struggling to say they don't need — the human value intrinsic within them outweighs all other consideration. Or it should do, if you're interested in health, mental health and peace-of-mind at that.

Bombing other human beings into smithereens cuts you off from the delights that they could supply you with. Be assured you cannot have peace-of-mind without *nutritious emotions* — and you cannot have *nutritious emotions* without living human beings. Reducing them to rubble along with their precious possessions also removes them from providing you and yours with invaluable mental treasures. Peace, as offered here, might sound impossibly costly — but, as they said about education — if you think education is expensive, you should try ignorance. Peace, in the form of white goods and other consumer aids is incredibly cheap, once you consider the alternative. *Roll on non-muddled thinking.*

'When I Meet Someone Without a Smile, I Give Them One of Mine'

IN CLOSING THIS CHAPTER, let's review the advantages of undoing *muddled thinking.* First off, we need to penetrate through the cloud of *scientism.* Over the centuries it became cemented into scientific thought that 'objective' was good, and 'subjective' bad. Poetry was fine, but since it wasn't scientific, it didn't really count. Occasionally, poets and other artists were allowed a 'deeper' truth, as if there were two varieties — one proper, and the other artistic.

The bargain was — forgo your individual views, your personal opinions, your very own feelings — and we'll eventually forge a *universal truth* that will supersede all others. All will be known, and all manner of things will be known. Well, it's a dream that failed. Just ask your favourite scientist whatever happened to the Higgs Boson? And if subjectivity is so taboo, how do they decide which of the two Hubble constants they personally feel most comfortable with? What is their personal preference? Or, since nothing moves without the electron, please could he or she tell you not only where a given electron is, but also, and at precisely the same time, where it is going? Explain, patiently, that you don't want *probabilities*, you want *certainties*. Science offered them, so why hasn't it delivered? Well it hasn't. And we need to get back to a deeper, a healthier realism.

Let's take another look at *truth*. I prefer a pragmatic definition — so truth in my book is the degree to which your picture, your model of the world that you currently inhabit reflects what is really going on outside. It can never be 100%. This is partly because we are fallible human beings and our senses and our reasoning are not limitless. But largely because the world out there may seem straightforward and patternful — but, in reality, the more we find out about it, the less it all makes sense. Much of the many papers on which this book is based go through chapter and verse to cement home this utter scepticism. Don't throw it all away, pick up the bits which make most sense, but don't expect a *universal answer*, a *single universal theory* which will let you off the hook — because there isn't one, and it won't.

But truth in this sense, matters. It matters more than life or death. Because, in common with all other living organisms that ever were, or ever will be, we need to respond to changes in our environment. If it gets too hot, we need to cool off, or too cold, to heat up — every single animal or plant that ever lived has to do this, else they cease to be alive. The Iron Law of Life is — adapt to your local reality, or perish. I didn't make this up, nor did you — but, since this book is based on a healthier view than the reverse, we need to stress it — be real, be realistic, be awake, else the opposite of health beckons.

Which is where *muddled thinking* costs. If your thinking is blocked, or diverted because of some faulty emotional education, then the penalty is not decreed by me, or by any other human agency — but by life itself. If you think there's enough oxygen in the room, because that's what you've always believed, or been taught — well let's hope there is, because, if there isn't, I don't have to tell you what'll happen.

Having restored the supremacy of what your opinions, your views, are, let's argue with them a little, let's open the windows a bit, to let in more light, and indeed more delight. One of the more tragic effects of friendless childhoods is that friendships don't count. Social skill, like any other skill, needs to be learnt. It is not always easy. Some humans can be really cantankerous. So let's have a look at why they shouldn't be.

I can't resist including here an 'answer' to the black hole that *science* leaves in our knowledge. It goes back to the *triple values*. I don't have eyes in the back of my head. I can see some things clearly, and others hardly at all. So how do I know that there isn't some evil creeping up from behind? Well, I ask around. I listen to what others have to say — if they see trouble, I listen and take action. If they reassure me, then the more reassurance I have, the better I will feel, and the more secure will be my peace-of-mind. Here is the mechanism behind no-one-is-sane-until-we're-all-sane. I need social contacts to stay sane. I need healthy, truthful contacts — and so, I would suggest, do you.

And here's the thing. When I see how others have solved some of life's challenges, I like it. Not only do I like it, but I take a delight in it. The very solving creates delight. I get great fun from trying to cajole words on a page to convey what I want them to — I delight in it. My aim is to delight you with it too — not that I can always guarantee success — but the very fact that I'm trying, helps.

Again, this tends to point to such complexity that the thread gets lost, it doesn't do what I want it to do — my verbal skills flounder. As before, get simple. Take a smile. What is a smile? Well, you could say it's the lips curling up at the edges. Or you could say, it really must extend to include the eyes. Or, even simpler, you could watch the next person who smiles at you — and enjoy it. Because that's what it's for.

And, miracle of miracles, if you give your smile away — you double it. You have more than you started with. This doesn't happen to physical objects. If you share your loaf of bread, you end up with half a loaf. However, if you share your smiles, you double them. Now this is an intrinsic bargain, available to every human ever born. It is, in my clear view, a human birthright. *Muddled thinking* might blank it into non-existence — but if you ever see a smile occurring, you should legitimately ask why you can't have one — because healthy social thinking determines that he or she can, and you should. You may have a stretch to go to the full extent of saying a-smile-a-day-keeps-the-doctor-away — but I have every expectation that you'll come to it.

And here comes the crunch. If you once shake off the shroud that has come to be attached to subjectivity, then what you feel, what you think and indeed what you decide, in your own mind becomes crucial. And what applies to you, also applies equally to me. My thoughts, conjectures, and imaginings matter too — but please note very carefully, I do not insist that the things I dream up are *right*, are the *one and only*, which I mandate on you to accept. *No*, I apply the triple values throughout — thus I request your consent to trust that

I will adhere to the truth as far as is humanly possible. And given what human endeavour can do, then that is not to be easily dismissed, either when I do it, or, gentle reader, when you do.

As we saw with the murderers, there is no scientific moral law which compels you or anyone else to do something, or to not do something—all we're left with is 'intent', the need for consent, to evaluate trust, so as to get as close to the truth as we possibly can.

Now, once this fluidity is established and universally agreed, then the converse immediately follows—this flexibility allows ingenuity, creativity and thereby delight, to flourish. What I like is legitimate. Provided I adhere to the triple values as tightly as I can, what I enjoy can be of interest to you and vice versa. What other humans do to solve everyday problems becomes intriguing. You have to stop second-guessing them—are they doing you down, are they operating on sinister and hidden motives, or do they genuinely demonstrate personal and friendly, indeed a social, interest in you?

So, we come to smiles. I smile when I'm pleased. If you're pleased to see me, then I welcome your attesting to this, by your smile. It goes right in. It bypasses words. And it matters. Thinking along these lines I came upon the phrase a-smile-a-day-keeps-the-doctor-away. When a friend of mine read this in my paper, he responded 'When I meet someone without a smile, I give them one of mine'—thereby demonstrating that a smile shared is a smile doubled. And when you take this that bit further, you begin to see more meaning in the notion that no-one-is-sane-until-we're-all-sane.

CHAPTER 3

Revenge Rots You

Nursery Nightmares — 'If Hitler Were Killing a Mouse He
Would Know How to Make it Seem Like a Dragon' — Daniel
Defoe Defies Revenge — Goodbye Yesterday's Nasties

Nursery Nightmares

ALEC DIDN'T LOOK LIKE A SERIAL KILLER. Admittedly, he had a tendency to sit on the edge of the chair, didn't smile much, and was certainly very intense. But he didn't roll his eyes or give you dark or evil stares like the typical Hollywood villain is supposed to. No, he looked what he was — an above-average intelligent man, fully capable of concentrating on a given task in hand, working out in careful detail how to do it, and then seeing it through to completion, with a dedication that would have been thoroughly admirable in healthier circumstances. It is surprising how much you can glean from first impressions. And what you can so easily miss, if that person doesn't want you to know. With Alec, the really remarkable thing is what his mother eventually saw in him, anew, when he'd finally purged his mental world of the hideous shadow which had dogged him all his life. Since the age of four. That verbatim paragraph alone, included later, justifies this whole excursion.

Sitting there, engaging in his first conversation with me, you can feel a decided reluctance on his part to talk at all. He agrees to do so, but only with half a heart. It's as if his mind is preoccupied, as if there are more important matters, which he can't deal with right now, but they lurk in the background like an evil, half-seen, threat. So how do I handle it? What's my technique? Where am I heading?

Well first, I try and open-up the conversation. After the initial preliminaries, I bounce things around, to see how flexible, free and easy he is. Do items come and go fluidly in his mind, like they should? Or is he especially guarded, when approaching emotive topics? Sure enough, as we skirt round more highly charged items, he tends to freeze up, he slows down, he gives out non-verbal cues that he's unhappy with that line of argument—an unspoken silent directive to change the subject. Which loudly indicates to me precisely where work needs to be done.

To be clear, I am not just having an afternoon's conversation. I am at work. My task is to find out where his rigidities come from, show them to him, and encourage him to bulldoze them out of the way. By this time, I knew I was looking for *muddled thinking*—I knew how to find it, and I was fast learning how best to rectify it. As his later escapade with throttling his pillow showed, I still had some way to go, but my confidence that there was real scope here was already strong.

We start with generalities. He has things to tell me about how he was determined not to come here, to this Special Unit, C-Wing (as it was called and existed at the time). He had heard dangerous things about it, and he armed himself so as to take violent steps to prevent himself being coerced into coming here. And it is certainly true that the regular inhabitants of this wing were generally deemed too violent for Broadmoor, the notorious prison 'hospital' for the insane. And stories had even come to my ears, that in earlier years there had been a murder here, one prisoner killing another. A story I could well believe, especially as one man later confessed that he would have killed three times here, had he not been talking to me—but that's another story.

And as Alec tells it, he so nearly didn't arrive. He told the prison officer admitting him in reception that he was determined to go down to the solitary confinement block right away. He resisted, as hard as he could, ever coming into C-Wing in the first place. No, it was not for him. 'Get me off this Isle of Wight'—he had said with considerable force. Happily, for him, and for me, he was being processed by an exceptional senior officer from C-Wing, a man I had had long and meaningful conversations with, as to what I was trying to do, and the way I was going about it. This man, let's call him Colin, saw where Alec was coming from, explained to him that he had no need to come and talk to me if he didn't want to—but, and here's the crunch, C-Wing was what he needed, and this was the reason he had been sent here.

There is Alec, carefully not telling me what's going on in his mind. Answering me, politely, with sparse information. What he didn't tell me, indeed it only came out much later, and even then, as an aside—when aged four, his father had thrown his mother down the stairs.

Bang—take yourself back into toddler-mode—what would it do to your mental world if one of the pillars of your very survival nearly killed the other one? Don't underestimate the damage. Aged four, you know that without parents, you are lost, you are over, you are finished. As before, titanic emotions attend all scenarios associated with life or death. Enormous quantities of treasure are invested in 'security', in 'defence'—why? Because you only die once, and while alive your emotions power you to do heroic things to defer it. That's what they're for. The human trouble is that powerful emotions tend to blur things—that's fine, if they allow you to prioritise escape, but less so if the threat is no longer real, but the effort you are expending is. Fighting ferocious phantoms can be lethal.

So here, hidden behind Alec's reticence, is a ghastly secret. Obvious enough when he was small, but fiercely buried ever since. Even to think about it, let alone verbalise it, would shoot Alec straight back into that scene where his mother is tumbling down, to her doom. Would you dwell on it? Why would you, when there was not a blind thing you, or Alec, could do about it? Aged four, you're small. Alec was small enough to be thrown out the window, let alone down the stairs—he could no more hinder his lethal father than fly.

Would you expect such a cataclysm to leave a residue? This is an explosion of emotions—if it didn't leave a mark, now that would be a surprise. What it does do, is bury the whole thing. If you can't do anything about it, *and* it's extremely painful even to turn it over in your mind—don't. Block it off, push it away, bury it behind anything else that comes to hand. It leaks out, of course. Bits of hostile feelings seep out into your everyday world—you cannot be entirely waterproof, not with something as huge as this. It rumbles on in the background, only half-seen. And yet it remains powerful. It will always be powerful, until you stop being four, until you grow to adult size, emotionally, and can remonstrate, successfully, with any lethal fathers who happen your way.

Meanwhile, your angry emotions have a field day. They are outside your everyday, conscious, rational control—but they haven't gone away. There's no limit to what excesses they may come up with. Indeed, once you tune into this sort of *muddled thinking*, the range of absurdities, of eccentricities is limited only by the human imagination — which, as you well know, has few limits.

In Alec's case, his anger against his father was redirected at other men. He couldn't shout at his dad — that would have been suicidal, and he'd learnt well and deeply enough to avoid doing that. In a distorted way, he killed his parental-figment, in lieu. This was something that emerged in every one of the other 50 murderers I worked with, that is once I had earned their trust. Killing came about because they thought they were about to be killed in the past, and they were taking revenge — not on the person who did it, they had been too small. No, on any substitute that offered itself in that person's place. In Alec's case this was other men — one every two years would satisfy the part of him that wanted to keep killing. For Putin, and other demagogues, their scope being wider, this means that the death toll is commensurately higher. Once you stop thinking straight, neighbours, especially in a next-door country, become prime unwitting targets, as the Ukrainians have found.

And why? Well in Alec's case it was his nursery nightmare. And this I have found to be the case wherever *muddled thinking* occurs. You can't go through the front-door. The way to talk things through is blocked. The nursery nightmare is still going on in their head — their mother is still tumbling to her death, their father is still doing unspeakable things, childhood catastrophes are continuing to happen, as we speak. Except they're not. You and I might well know that the nursery nightmare is well and truly in the past — but they don't, and they don't welcome you telling them. Have a care. The *truth* is deadly, as far as they are concerned, and shooting the messenger is by far the quickest way to escape an inevitable, highly lethal nightmare. Waking-up is a better remedy, indeed a cure, but that takes some believing.

'If Hitler Were Killing a Mouse He Would Know How to Make it Seem Like a Dragon'

OF COURSE, NURSERY NIGHTMARES leave many tell-tales. Once you are alert to them, they crop up all over the place. If we move away from Alec, and from Putin, back into recent history, then Hitler comes to the fore, and his story is poignant, relevant, and pungently bitter-sweet.

To my surprise, I came across an astute examination of what went on in Hitler's mind from a source I had not expected—George Orwell. In March 1940, a few months before the Battle of Britain finally put an end to Hitler's plans to invade the British Isles, Orwell published a literary review of Hitler's master work, *Mein Kampf* (see *Appendix 3*). I have numbered the extracts below for convenience:

'§5 But Hitler could not have succeeded against his many rivals if it had not been for the attraction of his own personality, which one can feel even in the clumsy writing of *Mein Kampf*, and which is no doubt overwhelming when one hears his speeches … The fact is that there is something deeply appealing about him. One feels it again when one sees his photographs—and I recommend especially the photograph at the beginning of Hurst and Blackett's edition, which shows Hitler in his early Brownshirt days. It is a pathetic, dog-like face, *the face of a man suffering under intolerable wrongs*. In a rather more manly way it reproduces the expression of innumerable pictures of Christ crucified, and there is little doubt that that is how Hitler sees himself. *The initial, personal cause of his grievance against the universe can only be guessed at; but at any rate the grievance is here.* He is the martyr, the victim, Prometheus chained to the rock, the self-sacrificing hero who fights single-handed against impossible odds. *If he were killing a mouse he would know how to make it seem like a dragon.* One feels, as with Napoleon, that he is fighting against destiny, that he can't win, and yet that he somehow deserves to. The attraction of such a pose is of course enormous; *half the films that one sees turn upon some such theme.*' (All emphases added by this author)

Bear in mind, this refers to the most dangerous man in the twentieth century, who was about to destroy Orwell's home, his way of life, his civilisation. Orwell sees, as clear as day, a deep and driving 'personal grievance'. He doesn't know where it comes from, but he is in no doubt that it is there. Orwell suffers least from *muddled thinking*—indeed, his clarity, as in his novels, is searing, and rather too close to the bone with respect to the dystopias he so accurately foresaw. Hitler himself, as I describe later, confirms the general theme put forward here—his 'grievance' came from his past, a past he too describes with shattering clarity, and here listed under the general heading *nursery nightmares*.

'A man suffering under intolerable wrongs'—what an apt description of so many of the murderers I worked with, including Alec. Neither he, not Hitler, could tell you what those 'wrongs' were—but the evidence that they hurt, both at the time they were inflicted, and throughout later adult life, is overwhelming—at least it is if you are prepared to see it. And, of course, it's true. Or more correctly—it was true.

If your father had thrown your mother down the stairs, or your parents had inflicted on you what Hitler's parents did on to him, you would have had no difficulty in labelling this an 'intolerable wrong'. Except of course, you would never volunteer to do so, as indicated above. This dark secret would remain carefully invisible for as long as you lived, in the absence of—wait for it—*nutritious emotions*, at least in my book.

So to the wonderful phrase 'If he were killing a mouse he would know how to make it seem like a dragon.' So succinct, so clear—but where does this come from? Why would Hitler not accept that killing a mouse is reward enough in itself? Why go way over the top and insist you are really a dragon-slayer, instead of being a useful rodent controller? In my book, it comes from his perception that he is fighting 'single-handed against impossible odds'. And that comes from? Well, it'll be no surprise that here I claim it comes from *toddler-thinking*. How else to characterise an insecure toddler? You make a big noise, because you have zero confidence you will be heard at all. And if unheard, you'd be overlooked, and if overlooked at two, you'd be dead. Parents keep you alive—but only if they want to, and they manage to convince you that they intend to. And hidden in there is the vital ingredient of *nutritious emotions*. It occurs to me that your body somehow decides that—if you're not going to be kept alive—why bother to put on height. Hypopituitarism might sound way out of order—but the pituitary gland, which does so much controlling, is intimately linked to all other bodily functions, including as here, to physical growth. Emotions link to reality via the pituitary. You might not believe this, you might not want to believe it—but if it's *true*, as I believe it is, then you may be missing something really vital.

And that something is the simple maxim we should all have learnt from Covid, i.e.—no-one-is safe-until-we're-all-safe. Daniel Defoe's most famous hero might have seemed to contradict this — self-sufficiency and all that — but did he?

Daniel Defoe Defies Revenge

ROBINSON CRUSOE IS OFTEN HELD UP as an ideal — especially it would seem in economics textbooks. Indeed, many have wished to emulate him from time-to-time, if only in fantasy, which could be hazardous. And indeed, Defoe himself punctures his own plot by telling us that suddenly there was a footprint in the sand. Hah! It wasn't an uninhabited island after all — other people were about; he just hadn't come across them. This rather dents the whole point of his self-reliance — like the rest of us, he could have had help, all along. Crusoe's appeal, and it is often surprisingly strong, carries its own seeds of contradiction. If only everyone were brought up to value everyone else, then *nutritious emotions* would be commonplace — you might even call that the contra-Crusoe approach — it also happens to be one of *my* favourites.

But Defoe earns a place in this book for an equally unexpected riff on *revenge*. In tales of derring-do, blood and guts, and high adventure, you commonly find vengeance playing a central role. Even Orwell, in his comment on 'half the films that one sees', hints at it. Indeed, vast tracts of Hollywood output, and its ilk, would be rendered meaningless, were mindless revenge omitted on the grounds that it didn't make sense, emotional sense — which it doesn't.

But give Defoe his due — in *The Life, Adventures and Piracies of the Famous Captain Singleton* (1720), we meet a ship's surgeon, a man called William Walton. Altogether an unusual man, William convinces the pirate crew *not* to go for revenge. This is especially unexpected, since pirates would seem to be motivated almost exclusively by distorted revenge — something which, in my view, powers all crime. Having gone marauding ashore, in a land Defoe mis-identifies as Ceylon, Singleton and his party are bested by a group of inhabitants who, among other things, hide in a hollowed-out-tree, out of gunshot range. They manage to spear a number of the pirates, which leaves the latter, as Defoe says, 'mighty warm'. Watch what happens next — it doesn't follow the conventional storyline (again my emphases):

'We had enough of Ceylon, though some of our people were for going ashore again, sixty or seventy men together, *to be revenged;* but William persuaded them against it; and his reputation was so great among the men, as well as with us that were commanders, that he could influence them more than any of us. They were *upon their revenge,* and they would go on shore, and destroy five hundred of them. "Well," says William, "and suppose you do, what are you the better?" "Why, then," says one of them, speaking for the rest, "we shall have our satisfaction." "Well, and what will you be the better for that?" says William. They could then say nothing to that. "Then," says William, "if I mistake not, your business is money [they were pirates]. Now, I desire to know, if you conquer and kill two or three thousand of these poor creatures, they have no money, pray what will you get? They are poor naked wretches; what shall you gain by them? But then," says William, "perhaps, in doing this, you may chance to lose half-a-score of your own company, as it is very probable you may. Pray, what gain is in it? and what account can you give the captain for his lost men?" In short, William argued so effectually, that he convinced them that it was mere murder to do so ...'

Defoe tells us that William, the hero of this episode (and of the book), is a Quaker and gives him 'thee and thou speech', among other things, to confirm the same. Here he empowers him to undo this revenge. He achieves this, by virtue of the fact that his reasoning carries undue (and uncommon) weight, as Defoe tells us — 'more than those of us that were commanders'. The logic, the healthcare-thinking, is clear enough — sadly too few can reliably rise to this standard of reasoning, this clarity, this level of thought, and still be trusted. 'You want money? Go where money is. You want to kill people? How does that help? It doesn't even ease your revenge.' 'Satisfaction' is a contradiction in terms which doesn't begin to cover your un-thought-through hatred — rather, in reality, it grows it.

Take a closer look at 'satisfaction'. As before, we may comfortably assume that human beings like doing some things, and dislike doing others. Some of these 'likes' predispose to health, and some don't. And since this book is health-based, let's look at revenge from that perspective. It is already clear that 'liking' war and destruction is unhealthy — so let's take a closer look at the role revenge takes, and how it works.

Time to revisit *toddler-thinking*. Once your inner mental world ceases to work in tandem with the real (adult) world out there, then discrepancies are bound to occur. You can no longer use your ineffable human capacity for thinking through your problems, because part of you, often a substantial part, is entirely wrapped up with toddler-aims, that is, with keeping authorities sweet, either mum and/or dad, or other authority-figures which happen along. Standing on your own two feet sounds lovely, but only for other people—your lot in life is cast in a different direction, and such delights are not for you. They are—but who are you going to believe?

Catching up into adulthood, emotionally, is not something *toddler think-ers* find easy. They get stuck. Like Alec, they see the world in one way, and as long as that's there, they let it dictate what they do, what they see, and indeed what they say. They haven't got the wherewithal to break out from their *nursery nightmare*. Indeed, part of their very own mental furniture is a make-believe world in which wonderful things happen, in direct proportion to the way they didn't in reality, back then.

Revenge is where past disasters hang a large ball and chain round your neck—*toddler-thinking* stops you seeing it, and the weight itself stops you walking upright. You are reduced to lugging it around with you for the rest of your life. Sadly, you've never met anyone reliable, trustworthy enough for you to consent to believe them. The message could not be simpler—revenge is toddler-based, and tends to remain so, until enough *nutritious emotions* come your way.

And because the emotional explosion is still rumbling on, as it was with Alec with respect to his father throwing his mother down the stairs—then revenge perpetuates itself. You keep adding to the damage you wanted to do to the original perpetrator, but can no longer—they aren't there anymore. So many others suffer, in their place—and, at each turn of the screw, your 'satisfaction' goes down, your need for revenge goes up, and your *nursery nightmare* is rein-forced, and cemented ever deeper in. You have been told the world is an awful place—so what's wrong with adding to what's already there?

If you have a better explanation for the thinking behind Hitler's 'Final Solution', then you'd better say so, and pronto, because there are too many look-a-likes just as driven as he was. *Nursery nightmares* might sound innocent—but cease to be so, when the person suffering from them is capable, powerful, and sometimes a commander-in-chief.

One final run-around on revenge. Say you broke my leg. By way of revenge I break yours. How does this help? The world would then have two cripples in place of one. Less *muddled thinking* would look for an adult-in-the-room (which requires adequate supplies of *nutritious emotions*), and then, using their good offices, the contention can be resolved, in precisely the same way teacher ensures that the local bully gives you back your favourite toy. Adults-in-the-room — sounds a bit like the legal system — the next chapter takes a closer look at how that might work better.

Goodbye Yesterday's Nasties

EMOTIONS! — Don't you just *love* them! — Don't you just *hate* them! Stop right there. Hold that thought. You have just solved one of the great human mysteries. A knotty philosophical or theoretical problem which has tied up more thinking time, and delivered more unhappy outcomes, than you could easily imagine. The solution lies in *not* asking what a feeling is — but ask rather, whether it is positive or negative. Is it encouraging or discouraging? Does it help you along, or hold you back? Is it more towards the 'love' end, or the 'hate' end? And if you don't know what those two emotive terms mean, perhaps you should get out more.

Earlier we simplified food by saying it's what went into the mouth. In some ways you might judge that to be oversimplification. But if you approach it with goodwill, with good intentions, then it offers enormous advantages. Exactly the same applies to emotions. They are what you react with. Sounds a bit awkward to put it like that. But then words are not the best way of describing feelings. Feelings are. It's like that litre (or pint) of water — suppose you insisted on only drinking 'square' water — well, you'd soon die of thirst. You'd perhaps feel a bit sorry for someone who insisted on defining the shape of their drink, before they drank it — it wouldn't make sense, it wouldn't add to the general wellbeing, or as in this book, to health. No, rigidity of definition can cripple, or worse.

And flexibility is called for, all over the place. Again, the lure of 'science' was that it would do away, once and for all, with woolly thinking, with variable definitions, with fluid notions — it would fix things for one and all. Any who insisted they wanted their water oblong, or spherical, would be firmly put in their place by being branded 'unscientific', and thereby beyond the pale.

The Greeks started it — they measured the side of a right-angled triangle, and to their delight it always came out the same ratio with the other sides. Wow, they thought, we're on to something here — just keep going, and we'll find the ratio for everything else in this complicated and apparently so chaotic world. It didn't take them long to find an exception — the world is riddled with them. Circles for example, just simply refused to comply. The length across was never an exact fraction of the distance around — technically, the radius has an unusual ratio to the circumference. The Greeks labelled this ratio π (Pi). They were so heartbroken, they scapegoated the number itself — calling it derisively 'irrational'. I once heard of a book that 'defines' π to a million decimal places. I fail to see the point of that — but once people get the bit between their teeth, there's no end to what they will come up with.

Let's accept that emotions are fluid. I'm happy to try describing them, but defining them once and for all just doesn't work. They seem to come and go, all by themselves. And a lot of the time they do. But, and here's the thing, if you can see where they're coming from, then you can nudge them, even put them entirely to rest. But look at that brief description just now — emotions are what you react with. You react to what happens. If you didn't, you'd be dead. Say the room gets overcrowded, and oxygen becomes scarce. What do you do next? Well, first you feel uncomfortable, and then you move, you do something, your emotions drive you along, even if you think otherwise.

Note that phrase 'feel uncomfortable'. Don't try defining it, but do pay attention to it. Because, if you don't, you're dead. Thus, emotions are reactions. Something happens, you either like it, or not. And depending on what 'value' you place on it, you either encourage it, or not. That's what having an emotion means — it's having a motion, a movement towards or away. See how easily you can fit all emotions onto a sliding scale — love at one end, hate at the other. Or, if you want to be more medical about it, positive emotions and negative ones — joy, delight, happiness versus anger, hate and fear. And the key, at least the way I've found it, lies in that last one — pull out the fear, and all the others fall meekly into place. You might have to see this to believe it — but I have seen it so often, I've even written a book about it.

55

It's so important to agree that emotions exist, even though we can never tell exactly what they are. The world doesn't take kindly to our 'scientific' precisions — it's vague, it's variable — and it can also be most exciting, even delightful. Once you acquire a level of verbal confidence, that's to say enough *nutritious emotions* to carry you forwards, then you can see how, despite being indefinable, a whole series of things can be discussed, sorted through, and indeed solved — goals that are simply unavailable if you keep fretting about what exactly 'fear' means, or 'anger'.

So how does *muddled thinking* come into all this? Well first of all the world out there is intrinsically muddled, even before we begin. That's to say, it doesn't, and never can make 100% sense. We have to make do with half-truths, lesser truths, bits of truth. And we have to exercise our judgment, our discretion, our responsibility — if we are to make any steady progress at all. The point I'm making is that health does occur — our task is to work out the best, if imperfect, way to ensure it does so to the best of our ability, yours and mine. And lurking always in the background, is war, which can never solve anything.

Muddled thinking makes no sense, unless you understand fear. The phrase once bitten twice shy, explains it. Alec found his father throwing his mother down the stairs so painful, he never volunteered to revisit it. It was over by the time I met him. It was 20 years in the past. But it was still alive in his head, his father was throwing her down every second, every micro-second. My task was to suggest otherwise. It sounds simple, but as events showed, it is also fraught.

We have a wonderful ability to remember — but why not concentrate on remembering the good bits, the positive end of the emotional spectrum? Of course, much of the time we can, and we do. Happy reminiscences make all the difference. But, and here's the thing — it's the heavies which do the damage. Some things must have happened in Alec's childhood that were fun — perhaps not many, but certainly some. So why did the worst of all stick longest. Not only stick, but closed the door on their own removal — on pain of killing the person trying to implement the removal. Quite a conundrum. Quite a deep root for revenge. And yet, these dreadful events are past, they are *not* operating in the present. However unsafe yesterday was, today is vastly safer by comparison. For one thing, you can walk about — you no longer need toddle. And, best of all for everyone, you can actually stand on your own two feet, not only physically, but emotionally too—and once you can do that 100%, then you can finally kiss yesterday's nasties goodbye, as Alec eventually did.

CHAPTER 4

Retribution Rots Judges

Thank Heavens for Nicaragua — Why Did Hitler Hit His Mother? — 'You're Brainwashed into Fear' — Vindication Perhaps, Retribution Never

Thank Heavens for Nicaragua

'AS A HIGH COURT JUDGE, I'M NOT THE LEAST BIT INTERESTED in why you hit women — so I'm sentencing you to live where there aren't any.' Can you see the *muddled thinking* here? Too few judges can. But put these words or similar into the mouth of a doctor, and the anomaly is glaring. 'As your doctor, I'm not the least bit interested in whether your chest pain comes from a heart attack, or not. Either way, I'm sending you to a holding bay, where follow up is unlikely.'

This cavalier medical approach would be quite unacceptable — why, we might even pass laws to curb it. But essentially the same happens every week, perhaps every day, in law courts all over the place. And all the while there is abundant evidence of where violence does come from, and indeed how to put it right. Violence against women in particular leads to so many deaths, it has earned its own label — femicide — horrendous, mindless, on a par with war, and just as soluble by clarity of thought.

Since we're now discussing what happens, or doesn't happen, in the court-room, it's as well to benefit from the invaluable insight which legal practice brings to the question of *truth*. You can't have sanity without clarity — and, since there's no longer any such thing as *absolute truth*, except in childish imaginations, it helps to be as realistic as we can about what we're left with. And in law, there are only two varieties of *truth*, one a higher standard than the other. There is — 'True, beyond-reasonable-doubt', and then — 'True, on a balance-of-probabilities'.

The advantage of this classification is that it's easy to grasp. Beyond-reasonable-doubt means what it says—you can doubt what I say is true, but if you're being reasonable then you have less grounds for doing so. Where truth is murkier, since there are infinite sources of doubt all around us, it makes sense to have a lesser variety—that's to say one where something is only 'probably' true (i.e. more likely to be true than not, that is on a balance of probabilities). Here reasonable men and women can differ, they can weigh up the different accounts, quite reasonably, and still not agree. Once the *uncertainty principle* holds sway, which it now does, all we're left with is *truths* which are more or less probable than any other. It takes a bit of getting used to—but there it is. And if you're interested in health, then reality adds that extra bite—without realism, you are unlikely to live as long.

Of course, the more cynical amongst us cannot resist adding that the one thing about life that is *absolutely true* is that we all die—but, since I've acquired a cheerful disposition, I prefer to leave that out of the equation, as long as I can. Let's move straight into philosophy, and consider the more theoretical aspects of the law. There have been calls to make legal affairs more 'scientific'. It sounds eminently sensible. Let's find out what the *scientific truth* is, then get a computer to enunciate it, so by-passing the human errors which too many judges (and legislators) fall into. If you can get computers to predict the weather, then why not the future of human behaviour? Especially when that behaviour goes off the rails, into crime?

Well, as many of my academic papers (see *Appendix 1*) set out to show, this is the Great Science Illusion—it doesn't hold water. What needs to happen is that *science* becomes more law-abiding, and thereafter follows every scientific statement with one or other of these two legal standards—saying, for example, 'Science shows, beyond-reasonable-doubt, that violence is curable'—or, for those still unaware, 'On a balance-of-probabilities—childhoods matter'.

In this sense, this book does not offer an irrefutable, *absolute, scientific* position—because there isn't one. No, it represents a prolonged medico-legal opinion—and you, gentle reader, have been enrolled as an all-important member of the jury. You may discuss with whomever you wish, in public, in private, on social media or elsewhere—but never doubt that your verdict is the one that matters. I'm putting forward the case against war, as I see it—your task is to adjudicate how true, or indeed how relevant that is to our present global predicament. Of course, I am free to use all the wiles that the best courtroom advocates avail themselves of. But equally, you have to be up to scratch, to spot the ones that are over the top, and only buy the ones which make most sense. Don't expect the question to be decided for you by anyone else—you have a mind, you can think, so do so. And let's hear your verdict loud and clear—that way we may all survive that bit longer—or can hope to.

Now you might object that no-one knows where violence comes from—so all you can expect from judges and the law is to stamp on it, whenever they see it. And of course, this can perfectly well be argued—but only if you point blank refuse to look at the abundant evidence. And you may also wish to rely on the conventional wisdom which says violent people are born that way, and there's nothing you can do about it. Again, you have to work pretty hard at keeping your eyes shut, or at least away from overwhelming evidence against such pessimism. Just because everyone else thinks violence is incurable, doesn't mean it isn't curable. It only means you're not interested in looking closely enough. Well, this book seeks to reverse that, and so we now need to travel to Central America, to the small, but important nation, Nicaragua.

Why Nicaragua? Well, it's a poor country, so it can't afford projects and services that are costly. More, if they can do it there, then rich countries have no excuse whatsoever—and if we don't implement what they did, we must, eventually, face up to the fact that it is not because we're unable, it's just another downside of our very own *muddled thinking*. What can Nicaragua tell us about violence? Well, outside researchers wanted to know how many women there had suffered physical violence from their partner. When they asked this in 1995, some 28% said they had. When they repeated the question, in 2016, this number fell to 8%—a more than three-fold reduction. When they then asked how many had never been beaten by a partner, the results were equally impressive. More than half had been hit in 1995—but this fell to only a quarter in 2016. All right, this meant that 25% were still suffering mindless partner violence—but look at the figures—if you had a 50% reduction in any disease you'd be over the moon and would ensure that everyone at risk could benefit. It's time we applied the same logic, the same thinking to violence. It's a curable disease and like smallpox should therefore be eliminated—if only we could think about it clearly. What else do you need a jury for?

61

So how did Nicaragua do it? I'm glad you asked. It wasn't ferociously expensive, else it couldn't have happened there. What did it need? It needed clarity of thought. It required thinking of women as equal citizens. And it absolutely demanded that we regard any, and all violence as not only sick, unhealthy, but eliminable. What they actually did, was to set up special police centres, well-staffed, readily available, with experienced doctors, counsellors, supporters — none of it rocket science — all eminently understandable, and covered here by the generic term *nutritious emotions*. Simple, but until it can get thought through clearly enough it is obviously far from easy.

You could argue that a doctor's obligation is to health, whereas a judge's is to uphold the law. But in this book that doesn't wash — health covers social health too, and there judges have a big and onerous role to play. All right, judges may claim that their hands are tied by what the law actually says — lawyers in my acquaintance 'read with their finger' — they follow the wording intently. But it is a poor, or sadly inexperienced judge who has yet to learn that the spirit of the law far outweighs the letter. Likewise, lawmakers need to open their minds wider, to ask, out loud — 'If Nicaragua can do it — what's holding us back?' And if they press that question far enough, as they certainly should, then *muddled thinking* comes to the fore, which is where I rest my case.

Why Did Hitler Hit His Mother?

HOW DO I KNOW THAT HITLER HIT HIS MOTHER? Well, because he says so, in his own words — his writing (see below) could not be clearer. Not only did he beat her, he was also sent to prison for doing so — and this gave him, as he puts it, 'his final polish'. If only the judge hearing his case had shown a little more interest in *why* he attacked his mother, the world could well be a safer place today. Social health might sound over-idealistic, but our concepts of society and its ills, does not wait upon our verbal niceties. The world around us does not owe us a living. If we fail to observe elementary health rules, we don't survive. This is so obvious from all the living creatures around us, that it's odd that it fails to penetrate our everyday thinking. Or rather, it would be, if we knew nothing about *muddled thinking*. Because it's here that *muddled thinking* takes its toll. We can dream up whatever we fancy — we're very good at that—it's when our thoughts and our words veer too far from reality that we come to grief. It's when *nursery nightmares* take precedence over harsh reality that disasters are inevitable. And the way to stop such nightmares starting in the first place is to conjure up enough *nutritious emotions* to prevent them—but, like all emotions, these struggle to gain acceptance, being intrinsically woolly, if delightful.

Mein Kampf (My Struggle) was written by Hitler in 1925, when he was 36. He had been sentenced to prison again, this time for leading an insurrection in which people were killed. He spent his time dictating his book. In it, as Orwell noted, he sets out his plans for domination—or, as I would put it, for misguided revenge for his appalling upbringing. In some places and at various times, the book itself has been declared illegal, hoping that the power of the law would somehow rinse away its evil—if people couldn't read it, they wouldn't be infected by it. A naïve view, which demeans human intelligence, and turns out to be a poor defence against the *toddler-thinking* you can so easily find there.

As a medical student, you are adjured to pay attention to any and all information or data that can help you understand where the disease in front of you is coming from. Because, obviously, the more accurate your diagnosis, the more your prescription is likely to improve matters rather than not. 'Listen to the patient, he or she is telling you the diagnosis' is my favourite clinical aphorism—it comes from William Osler, a highly insightful clinician, and it has saved my bacon on a number of occasions. Here, we look in Hitler's writings, where he describes why he set out to destroy the world—and did so so effectively we still suffer from it today. Worse, if we don't understand him, how can we possibly avoid inviting him and his ilk, back, for a repeat performance, at our terminal expense?

The other day, I was discussing with a paediatrician how childhood influences governed so much of adult life—and she confirmed that, as she put it, she tried to intervene 'before the child was broken'. A telling phrase, which prompted me to ask her if she knew that Hitler had been strapped to a chair as a child. She didn't. To double check this fact, I re-read Alice Miller, that wonderful pioneer into adverse childhoods, since, as I remembered it, that was where I had read this appalling fact. In the time available, I couldn't find it. But what I found was even more impressive—a page and a half of explicit prose, written by Hitler about his own upbringing, and describing in blood-curdling detail precisely why he later behaved as he did (the emphases are mine):[2]

> '§8. As he begins the more demanding parts of his life, *he falls into the ruts he has learned from his father.* He wanders about, comes home Heaven knows when, beats the tattered creature who was once his mother, curses God and the world, and finally he is sentenced to a prison for juvenile delinquents.
>
> §9. Here, he gets his final polish.'

Who would have thought that Hitler disapproved of imprisonment? Yet here he is, in his own words, condemning the treatment he received as a youth — 'his final polish' is indeed ominous. Do judges, and the lawmakers who write the laws, really know that this is actually what happened in the early years of the last century, just prior to the destruction of the world as we know it?

Let's suppose that, instead of a 'final polish' into destructive violence, he had been given enough *nutritious emotions* to head off his inherent revenge — what then? Is that really too fanciful? If social policy, and policing, can cut domestic violence by half, in one of the poorest countries in the world — what are we waiting for? Orwell was unaware of the appalling circumstances prevailing in Hitler's childhood — we have no such excuse. Every teenager we, and our judges, send to prison today, serves to bottle up revenge. And it's this revenge, thereafter applied also to 'the system', that powers a later life of crime, an aborted career, or, with demagogues, war.

Let's have some joined-up thinking. Social frictions are symptoms of deeper social disease. They need noting, they need paying attention to, they need curing at source — prevention here being so much cheaper than cure. I can't resist reviewing a recent policy statement by the then UK Prime Minister. He was responding to a particularly gruesome child murder. He promised to pursue all responsible and bring them to justice. What he would have found, had he really looked, was that his Government had systematically starved social services of funds, to the extent that these early symptoms, though detected, were met with grossly inadequate resources. How many troubled families would you

---

2.   For the full passage from *Mein Kampf* see *Appendix 3*. I have numbered the paragraphs for ease of reference. Additional commentary can be found in Johnson, 2022b (see *Appendix 1*).

like on *your* caseload? Every domestic fracas you are involved in takes its toll, inevitably—we are all human, we need social support too, especially when trying to head off worse. Cut funding for social support for 12 years, and it's no surprise that social diseases fester. Only when it is more generally accepted that no-one-is-safe-until-we're-all-safe, that social frictions can be eased by adequate social interventions—then the elimination of violence will be seen to be of value, and so to be worth paying for, by all.

Back to Hitler. As you read through these pages from *Mein Kampf,* the facts hit you in the eye. Of his parents, he says:

> '(§5)—'*They never utter a good word about humanity.* No institution is safe from their profane attacks, from the schoolteacher to the head of the state. No matter whether it is religion or morals, state or society, everything is defamed and dragged in the muck. When the boy leaves school at the age of fourteen, it is hard to tell which is greater—his incredible stupidity where common knowledge and basic skills are concerned, or his biting disrespect and bad manners. (Emphasis added)

> (§6) The immoral displays, even at that age, make one's hair stand on end.'

Here you have one of the most immoral people in the world, showing horror at his initial exposure to the denigration of 'morals'. One may dispute what morals or ethics really are, what, in essence, the Good Life is. But here is a display of revulsion at immorality—not what you might have expected, but there it is in black and white, obvious enough to all who are prepared to see.

The upshot, unsurprisingly, is that he concludes (§7) that:

> 'He holds almost nothing sacred. He has never met true greatness, *but he has experienced the abyss of everyday life.*' (Emphasis added)

If we cannot learn from the mouth of the most destructive man of the last 100 years—when can we learn? Are we all agreed that *everyday life* can never amount to more than an *abyss*? Is that really all we have to offer after millennia of civilisation? If you were taught that life was abyssal, then you may not raise an eyebrow that Hitler, too, was taught the same. However, there are those who say parts of life can be delightful. That interacting with other living human beings can bring joy, or at least, smiles. Democracy is rule by the majority—but, surely, we can lift our corporate eye above such an abyss, and aim for better? *Nutritious emotions* might seem too diffuse, too idealistic, and a bit of a struggle to come to terms with mentally—but however uphill, these verbal difficulties are molehills, compared with war.

'You're Brainwashed into Fear'

THE ROSETTA STONE WAS CARVED IN 196 BC. Once 'discovered', it transformed our knowledge of Ancient Egypt. Before Rosetta, Egyptian hieroglyphs were just an inscrutable sequence of the occasional bird intermingled with a scattering of intense human eyes, alternating with, and strung together by a whole series of squiggles—no-one knew what they meant, since no living soul remembered them. What the Rosetta Stone did was write the same message in both hieroglyphs and Greek—and since the latter was well known, the former became open to all. What's the connection with this book? Well, *muddled thinking* was equally unintelligible—it seemed to come out any which way up, making no sense either to the sufferer or to those hoping to help. The 'guff' given out by tyrants, killers and demagogues can be quite elaborate—but none of it adds up, at least not sufficiently to shine a light on how best to improve it.

And of course, as Alec showed, if you pursue the childhood issue too openly, then you join the abuser, the torturer, the problem, and cease to be of any help in resolving matters. So that was the issue—how do you get someone to tell you the last thing they want to tell themselves. Let's be quite clear about this—the trauma we're talking about was huge—big enough to freeze any further consideration of the event which had precipitated it. A closed loop was set up. Being small, there was nothing the child could do at the time—lethal dads or mums were not to be 'answered back'—you'd only try that once, and never again, far too risky. The odds were heavily against—your opponent was at least twice your size—and no-one in their right mind would tackle a 12 foot (four metre) high grizzly bear, emptyhanded—well only once.

And there's the issue. Ask the traumatised victim to tell us what the trouble was, and you immediately evoke it. You land them straight back into the original disaster scene, as if nothing had changed. It's called 'retraumatisation', and it can be deadly—either of you or of them.

No wonder today's psychiatry sees psychiatric symptoms as so many incoherent hieroglyphs—but that's another story, for another book altogether. Here we need a flavour of the mind going wrong, perhaps with the muddling just beginning to unfurl. A glimpse into how the illogic starts. The upshot is that the reasoning that is then in full flood, being non-verbal (as it with Ethan in *Chapter 2*), continues in the same *toddler flavour*. Nothing has happened to change it. The real tragedy, apart from all the mayhem, is that only one simple thing needs to happen—the sufferer needs to wake from their *nursery nightmares*—simple, but too often very far from easy.

Let's take a clip from my breakthrough dialogue with Lenny (see *Appendix 5*). Lenny's thought-blockage is telling his mother he is an adult. He had been far too terrified to even consider the idea. Watch carefully how Lenny gradually accepts more and more of my support, to address what up to that point had been his all too lethal fears. By confronting them, he calms them. They then evaporate, 100%.

'Line 37. Bob: Do you find that surprising, that you find it difficult to tell your mother you're an adult?

L38. Lenny: Yes. Very surprising.

L39. Bob: It is, isn't it? So what will stop you? Say your mother was sitting over there, what would you say to her?

L40. Lenny: I'd say "Mother you can't hit me anymore. I am an adult."

L41. Bob: And you believe that?

L42. Lenny: Yes. *Partly.*

L43. Bob: You partly believe it and partly don't?

L44. Lenny: Yes. I don't know whether I could say it to her or not.

L45. Bob: What would stop you?

L46. Lenny: Fear.

L47. Bob: Fear of what? What is she going to do?

L48. Lenny: Well she might get up *and clout me.*'[3]

---

3.   Here and elsewhere in this book where I set out dialogue with offenders the lines are taken from my professional notes/recordings, made at the time. Fuller extracts from 'Lenny's Dialogue' appear in *Appendix 5*.

Look at line Lines 39 and 40. I offer him an open invitation — what would he like to be able to say, if she were in the room with us both. And see how, in his response, he immediately adds his adulthood as being a (hitherto unavailable) defence against her ever hitting him again. This, at last, shows him the way to overturn his long-ago trauma.

Being an intrepid explorer, I challenge him on just how strong his new courage is. And being an honest broker (and trusting me implicitly) he confirms my suspicion that he only 'partly' believes it. To you or me, the question does not arise — he is an adult, and he has been for some three decades — *but not* in his own mind. And since being battered to death by an irate (if small) mother has lodged, like an abscess, in his private mental world, he was unable to move forwards. He didn't trust authorities, parental or police, since they had always let him down. And there was no point in discussing his terrors with someone weak, who would be equally cowed, and as easily overwhelmed. What he needed was someone powerful, *but also safe.* Not an easy combination to come by, especially as you would be asking for help for coping with the last thing you would ever admit, either to yourself or to anyone else.

'Hello, I'm 6 feet 3 inches [190 cms] — but I need reassurance that I'm an adult.' Who would you possibly ever admit this to? But until you did, as Lenny was able to, to me, then you're stuck with a crucifying conundrum — adult responsibilities coupled with only infant sized capabilities. No wonder, once established, *muddled thinking* self-perpetuates.

And look how critical *nutritious emotions* are. Lenny, by this time, trusts me. I am therefore able to deliver gentle encouragement. I feed his adult mind and wean it from its past impediments. *Truth, trust* and *consent* are therapeutic. This dialogue was recorded on 11 September 1991, only ten weeks after I arrived at Parkhurst, on 1 July 1991. It had taken me that long to reinstate my custom of videoing every consultation, where I could obtain consent.

The next time I showed it was to a room full of 100 psychiatrists, at their annual conference. I had to pinch myself while doing so — was I really talking to so many? You could have heard a pin drop. At the end, the ebullient president bounced down the aisle saying loudly, 'We have power, we can help'. I had mentioned there were ominous signs that the Government was about to close the Special Unit — and this vigorous offer of support was in response to that. Unhappily, that was the last I heard of it — my invitation to organize a session the following year was quietly suffocated, and much the same happened to what I judged to be a breakthrough in understanding why minds went wrong, what it was that really troubled them, and indeed, what steps could be taken to put it right. Within 18 months the unit was ignominiously closed

Lenny however, remains my star. A remarkable man. How many patients could say, as he did?:

'Line 231. That's right yes, but it's the truth, isn't it? The truth's got to come out hasn't it? And you were trying to help me, and I am helping you.'

What a wonderful endorsement of *truth*, as seen from the sufferer's end. Also, look at the confidence he has, and the joint enterprise we have set up. There is simply no doubt in his mind that, while I am helping him, he is unquestionably helping me. Which he certainly was, because by November 1991 he was out the other end and needed no further coaching from me. Others showed no change after two full years. Lenny not only enthusiastically supported what I was trying to do, but understood it at least as well as I did, and vastly better than most of the psychiatrists I have ever shown it to, including that full annual conference I've mentioned.

This is so close to my heart that I could carry on page after page, but doing so would undoubtedly stretch the patience of the jury, so I must, reluctantly, restrain myself. However, I will allow myself a few more lines of the dialogue, since they show how *muddled thinking* can be cured, and I do mean cured. Since this approach specifies that *muddled thinking* comes from a long-ago trauma, currently festering today, and in need of excision, my technique, to show no further intervention is needed, is to re-expose the person to what terrified them, speechless, before. In our November 1991 session, I ask Lenny what he would do if his mother came to hit him today:

'Line 256 Lenny: If this had've happened years ago, where a doctor had taken an interest say when I was in my twenties and said what you'd said and *we'd conquered it* [none of this would have happened].
L 257 Lenny: And then I went to the house. And say I came in late, and she said blah blah blah *and she went to hit me*, I'd say mother you can't hit me love — I'm a grown up. You can't do it. You can kick me out of the house

> L 258 Bob: Because it's your house
>
> L 259 Lenny: But you can't hit me — don't try and hit me
>
> L 260 Bob: But you've never said that up until the last month or two
>
> L 261 Lenny: Yes. I've never had the *confidence* to say it.
>
> L 262 Bob: That's right.
>
> L 263 Lenny: *You're brain washed into fear* ... [continued]'

Can I suggest to the jury, that undermining social confidence is precisely what happens in our Criminal Justice System? And that this is the last thing our police, and our courts, indeed our entire Government should have as their ongoing priority, which should be directed at building up confidence not the reverse.

Vindication Perhaps, Retribution Never

'LET'S BRAINWASH ALL OUR CRIMINALS INTO FEAR.' This adaptation of Lenny's Line 263, is a brilliant summary of how we currently run our so-called Criminal Justice Systems. It's an expensive way of making things worse, just like war. The jury will not be surprised to note that it is also a first-class demonstration of classical *toddler-thinking*. Suppose for a moment, that you were in charge of a feisty kindergarten, and you elected to run it on this basis — terrify your toddling charges into submission — anything for a quiet life. You could then report to your employing authority that you had managed to restore peace and quiet, or in the prevailing political mantra — law and order. And indeed, as the Gestapo proved, it does quieten things down — you get far less trouble, if you shoot all the troublemakers, or terrify them into submission.

And, let's face it, as the old saying has it — the prospect of being hung concentrates the mind remarkably. Which, as mentioned earlier, is precisely what fear is for. If, as suicide bombers prove all too often, you aren't frightened of getting killed, then there's no limit to what you will do. And as also mentioned, powerful emotions drive you forcibly — they take over — that's what they're for. Wake up, they say, stop whatever you're doing, and scarper. Why bother to think things through, when the house is on fire? Think, and you're dead. Time is of the essence. Those who indulge in wondering why, or in asking questions about longer-term impacts, or show unconcern about incurring future expense—they don't survive, so they don't offer a tempting alternative. The prospect of following their example is, frankly, unattractive.

My advice to you, gentle reader, is that if your life is currently in danger, close this page, and make for the exit, if you can find one. However, on the optimistic assumption that you are sitting comfortably, that your evening meal is assured, and you've a comfortable bed for the night, then please do put fear aside, and take a long cool look at what's at stake here. First *toddler-thinking,* then Lenny.

All well run kindergartens have adequate resources, plenty of available adult time, and (the main theme of this book) floods of *nutritious emotions.* Put yourself back into the toddler position, and you'll soon know what *nutritious emotions* are—they are smiles, cheerful comments, encouraging remarks—'You're doing well today, that was a lovely drawing you just did, what a clever little girl or boy you are.' Please use your fertile imagination to add your own positive phrases—I don't really need to define what *nutritious emotions* are in scientific terms—since like anyone else who has ever been a toddler, given the chance, you can generate a fruitful stream of them, all by yourself.

What I do need to do is re-emphasise quite how vital these friendly emotions are. And I use the word vital, advisedly. It may be painful to have to admit it, but toddlers grow better when you smile at them, and remain stunted when you scowl, or sneer. Yes, you can measure food and calories, and also inches and centimetres—so there's no difficulty in seeing how these progress under favourable childhood circumstances. Scientific measurements are rated very highly, so when they show that deficient emotions lead to deficits in measured physical size, you'd expect, indeed hope, that the role feelings play in maturation would be established without demur. And of course, sentient members of the jury will have no difficulty in accepting that favourable childhoods breed peaceable adults. Why wouldn't you?

But we need to press this further. Not only physical maturation, but cognitive progression too. If your infancy was dominated by fear, brainwashed in Lenny's phrase, as his was, then this stops you thinking. It prevents you moving on from *toddler-thinking* to a realistic, or a more adult, version. And indeed, as applies precisely to the case in point—if you were 'controlled' by fear, then you will 'know' that that's how things work. Naughty boys, and girls, behave—but only because they're frightened of what happens when they don't. The naughtier they are, the harder they need to be hit.

Which has the unhappy consequence — the more pain, the more fear, the less reflection, the less the thought. And so, we come to the rational explanation of 'guff' from *Chapter 1*. Fear drives out thought. When you ask a murderer why she/he killed, you get lots if illogic, as you do with the Supreme Court of the United States. It doesn't add up. Or rather, it doesn't add up in the real world — but it makes perfect sense for a toddler. When others are in charge of your life, then make sure you don't upset them, else that'll be the end of you. Only when you are responsible for what happens to you next do you take better care, either of yourself, your fellows, or indeed your world. *Toddler-thinking* costs.

At this point in the proceedings, in order to help the jury adjudicate, I would wish to bring in my star witness, Lenny. He responded to my approach within five months — others took far longer, so without his help I would never have been able to tackle such as Alec with sufficient confidence. I'll put Lenny on the stand, and ask him to explain just how fear brainwashed him — or, even more importantly how *nutritious emotions* restored his thinking. Unhappily I'm prevented from producing him. He is not available. For all I know he may even be dead. His mistreatment at the hands of the Prison Service, especially the prison psychiatric service, is something I'd love to investigate, if I ever had the authority. But, just as the then UK Government closed down my Parkhurst work, without trace, so they have consistently denied me access to my earlier clients. Which means we must press on without him in person, and we will have to make do with his verbatim comments.

Accordingly, look at Lenny's Line 261 above — my emotional support has assisted him by giving him *confidence*. This is what *nutritious emotions* are for. He was able to see that his earlier brainwashing prevented him telling his mother the *truth*, that he was an adult. Nothing remarkable, nothing vengeful — just today's reality — he was now as big in his mind as he was in body — his *toddler-thinking* was over.

What would be Lenny's message to the Criminal Justice System? You need only look at his Line 256 which I set out on its own below:

'If this had've happened years ago, where a doctor had taken an interest say when I was in my twenties and said what you'd said and *we'd conquered it* [none of this would have happened].'

Not only can Lenny now think straight, he can see so clearly that what we had done was not rocket science — it wasn't over the moon — it was something which could easily have been made available. Had it been, he would not now be serving a life sentence (if still alive), from which he is never likely to be released. A case of prevention being rather cheaper than cure.

So back to the High Court judge's utter disinterest in where violence comes from. The law is built, in this case, on *toddler-thinking*. Revenge is laid down in the Statute Book. Judges are condemned to increase it, not refute it. Retribution comes from the Latin 'pay back'. It means you hurt society, so we'll hurt you. It couldn't be a clearer example of misreading behaviour — or rather of *muddled thinking*. Something that can afflict even the highest court in the land — in a word — guff.

CHAPTER 5

Consent Empowers: But Bullying Others Saps You

'Head-Start' Paid for Itself: So Why Cut Funds for 'Sure-Start'? — 'I Consent Therefore I Am' — The Parental Dilemma — Consensual Delights

'Head-Start' Paid for Itself: So Why Cut Funds for 'Sure-Start'?

TODAY, DO YOU WANT TO PLAY WITH THE SAND AND WATER, or with the bricks? I don't know about you, but sand fascinates me — or it did. There was a time when watching how sand pours out the bucket — just like water does — was totally absorbing. I could watch it for ages. But then again, you can also build it up, ever so high — sandcastles have an appealing way of bringing out the builder in you. Aged two, I could spend many an afternoon building it up, and then starting all over again. Couldn't you? Or have you forgotten what it was like to be a toddler?

Perhaps all today's heavy 'adult' burdens currently weigh you down, pushing the happy days of yore out of your mind. Or, worse, perhaps you never had any to remember. When you were two years old, were you fortunate enough to be offered options, choices? Was it ever up to you, which of a range of delightful things you could do next? Or not?

OK, let's move the age range up to five, so we'd have a better chance of recall — but the question remains — how much was your opinion sought then? What turned on your decision, if anything? Well, since the running theme of this book is that childhoods matter, let's draw on some good solid scientific evidence. And, whether you can bring yourself to believe it or not, there is irrefutable, high quality, objective data readily available, to prove exactly this point — at least, as with all things scientific, there is — but only for those prepared to take a look.

Science means sorting through a selection of facts and theories, with the objective of finding the best way forwards. Nothing wrong with that—indeed it's the best way to proceed. Two factors, however, impede its sovereign progress—one, there isn't a definitive solution for all time, the world out there keeps changing all by itself, and even if you did manage to capture most of the *truth* today, the inherent chaos out there would ensure that by tomorrow, it would be out of date. Hard to accept, painful to have to admit—but there it is—what you know now is partial, it can never be 100% because, like it or not, time goes by, and even a few microseconds on the reality in which you live and breathe has changed. Hopefully it still has enough oxygen for you to breathe with—but there's no guarantee, only a strong probability—aided or obstructed, by your ability to observe, to think, and thereby to optimise, or degrade, your continuing strategies to keep alive and healthy.

The second flaw in *science* is believability. Even when the facts do add up, and the data does point decisively in one direction, you still find obstinate people trudging steadfastly and determinedly against. Contrary to popular wishful thinking, two things have gone wrong with science. Not only is there no *unique universal scientific theory* to ensure there is *only one line*, which commands attention and unthinking obedience from everyone, regardless. Secondly—even the solutions that do survive, whether only on a balance-of-probabilities basis or not, can be buried—they cut no ice, convince no waverers, and are dismissed as easily as yesterday's stale air. Ah, these humans, what can you do with them?

If the people in charge of your childhood gave you no evidence that childhoods matter, how can you be expected to differ? Well, because you can think for yourself—at least that's what your frontal lobes are for—working out whether Plan A is more likely to succeed than Plan B—and in this book, of course, better means healthier. And, in particular, to re-think. If the first way through isn't working—have you enough thinking ability to see this, to reconsider, and then launch in a new, and hopefully more up-to-date, more realistic, direction? Or not? Our global health depends on nothing less.

We're never going to get anything resembling a *totalitarian scientific view*. Not only will there always be exceptions, deviations, anomalies, where even the most fundamental building blocks are riddled through and through with *uncertainty*—not an easy truth to swallow, as Einstein found. But even where evidence does come close, you find people wilfully ignoring it, carrying on as if it had never been uncovered—indeed, reacting almost deliberately contrariwise. Climate change is a case in point. But here we're putting childhoods centre stage. Let's compare one sort of childhood with another. Let's look at which produces the best outcome, the best adult—Version One, or Version Two.

Well, you might think, every child is different, just as no parent is ever 100% the same as any other—so how can you investigate the quality of one type of childhood over another? But it has been done. If you can summon enough objectivity, put aside all those doubts, and take another, dispassionate look—why not see how 'Head-Start' works out?

In the USA in 1965, in an effort to tackle poverty, a trial scheme was set up. Careful thought was given to how to tell whether what you did to children, mattered—not only in the short-term, but over the decades. It was called 'Head-Start'. And what was special about it was that it divided the children it was dealing with into two carefully matched groups—Group One, and Group Two.

In Group One, the children were offered conventional play groups, say three afternoons a week. In the other, a type of super-playschool. I don't have the textbook in front of me, but the point about Group Two was that the child was put at the centre of things—hence the opening question of this chapter. What the child did was decided by the child. You could call it child centric, if you don't mind verbal shorthand. What happened next made all the difference—each child, from either group, was followed up, to see what happened to them in adult life—exceptional, unusual and quite remarkable.

And the difference in outcomes between the two groups was staggering. In the second, there were fewer marital breakdowns, more job security, less prison. In fact, the taxes paid by this group outperformed the other—to such an extent that the extra earned paid for the entire scheme itself. It actually pays, in hard cash, to give toddlers choice. If you do, they cost you less over the long-term. In Group Two, their additional confidence, self-esteem and better social skills enabled their work input to cover all the expenses of the scheme. You might call it investing in our future—children today become citizens tomorrow.

At that time, my particular interest was in psychotic symptoms, so when the then director of the scheme came over to the UK I pressed him to say whether there was less psychosis in Group Two. He was reluctant to agree—but I cheerfully assumed that that was because it wasn't in the data, not because mental health had failed to benefit.

As its name suggests, it really did give the selected children a 'Head-Start'. And it's as scientifically based as you can get. Which is why I find room for it here. It also makes so much sense — children are impressionable. If you treat them right, they'll behave right. Treat them badly, and you have only yourself to blame. Can we wake up in time?

Let's run a few of our example childhoods through the scheme. Suppose, aged three, Hitler had been given a different reference point. If, instead of being taught that life was abyssal, he had been educated to take delight in exercising his options, taking control of the events immediately around him, at least to the extent you can, at that age. It would then be inconceivable that he would have continued to work on the basis that life was an abyss — into which he could pour himself and everyone else. It stands to reason. It is also as near scientific proof as we can get.

Take Alec. Had he been cherished, even only three afternoons a week, then the change in his outlook inflicted on him by his father's lethal brutality to his mother would have manifested itself unmistakably, to outside observers. Sensible social support would then have been called for, and in civilised societies made readily available, such that several lives would have been saved, including, potentially, mine.

Lenny too, would have found healthier ways to deal with his fear of his mother. It was only decades later that he found that the missing ingredient in sorting out his mental furniture was 'confidence'. If the foundation stones for this had been laid when he was five we would all have benefited from his honesty, his fortitude, his persistence — just as I did, in 1991.

'Head-Start' was imported into the UK under the name 'Sure-Start', in a valiant attempt to improve social health, increase domestic stability, reduce criminality and result in more being paid in Government taxes for doing so, to say nothing of seeking to obviate war — what else are governments for? Unhappily 'Sure-Start' fell fall foul of the change of the UK Government in 2010 — as blatant an example of illogical *toddler thought* as you could dread. But enough of *science* for now — let's return to the emotions behind 'unbelievability', i.e. towards a healthier philosophy.

'I Consent Therefore I Am'

ONE DAY IN THE 1620s, René Descartes was sitting by his French stove. He was wrestling hard with perhaps the most complex problem of them all—so it wasn't really surprising that he goofed. It's important to be clear what he was trying to do, and why he failed. If we can learn from his mistakes, we'll all gain. He was musing on what thinking really meant—and, in particular, where consciousness came from. He'd already made substantial progress in how we think of things mathematically, his original concepts are still in regular use today—but being alive had him foxed. As he sat there, alone, it occurred to him that what distinguished him most from, say, a lump of wood was his ability to think. He coined the phrase 'I think, therefore I am'. He voiced this in Latin, which nowadays is less prevalent than it was—*cogito-ergo-sum*—I cogitate therefore I exist.

Sadly, for him, and for the many who still subscribe to his views, life, and indeed the world in which we find ourselves, does not take kindly to over-simplification. There are indeed *truths,* some of which do hold better than others—but none is ever 100%, as discussed in earlier chapters. However, thinking is a crucial, indeed a vital aspect of humans—so he was right there. What he failed to add in are the emotions. In this omission he is joined by far too many, who really should know better. Emotions trundle around as if they own the place—which in emergencies, they rightly do. But even in calmer periods, they play an indispensable part.

A phrase that comes to mind links the two together—there is no thought without an emotion—and no emotion without a thought. It doesn't always hold good, but it's better than basing your philosophy on thought alone. Emotions, as mentioned, add meaning—without them, things tend to become meaningless. What matters is controlling them—and the only way to do that is firstly to acknowledge they exist. Next, learn to understand them. And then ask where they come from, and what they're doing, both to you and your thoughts.

In July 1960, I was trying to capture some of this complexity in a book I chose to call *The Elusive Horizon* (Johnson, 1960, unpublished), so I remember having fun with the Latin, as follows: instead of *cogito-ergo-sum*, I tried *dormio-ergo-absum*—'I sleep, so I don't exist'. During a university lecture two years before, one which still sticks in my mind, I'd been shown how to tweak Descartes. That lecturer was talking about Sartre, another French philosopher—who, so he said, had reversed this significant phrase to read—*sum-ergo-cogito*—'I am, so I can think'. He explained that this is what the existentialists had done—they put 'existence' first, which is certainly healthier.

But back to the emotions. OK, they can never be defined, and will always remain defiantly subjective—it's what you feel, what you emote, what 'moves' you. As before, some are good, and some rather less so. So how should this impact on Descartes? How about adding them in to his phrase—'I think, and I have feelings—therefore, I exist'. A bit cumbersome, but at least it's moving in the right direction.

Take a tip from Sartre, and prioritise 'existence', and, bingo, you come up with 'health', at least I do. 'I think, so I can remain alive longer.' Or, contrariwise, 'thoughtlessness kills'. Word play like this can help, but it shouldn't distract from the seriousness of life, or of health which promotes it.

So why did I go to some trouble to call my first book *The Elusive Horizon*? Well, it was meant to capture, in three words, the reason 'science' could never succeed. In order to understand something, we first need to simplify—we can't swallow huge chunks of info all in one gulp—in technical terms, the input channel to thought is small—perhaps five or six novel items are manageable, but throw too much in at one time, and the thing gets clogged—'You lost me there, I fail to follow the thread, I don't understand what you're talking about.'

And, naturally, I had been thoroughly schooled in how *science* progressed from Mediaevalism, via sorcery and superstition, through to glorious rationality, in which behind everything was a reason, which time and effort could be relied on to reveal—provided we kept at it. I had done well in my science exams, and I had had an especially good grounding in the basics of physics and chemistry. But, alongside this confident striding forward, there was a persistent thread, which questioned the whole project. Doubt had been planted, in particular by a Scotsman, David Hume, who warned, in 1739, that all our knowledge was threadbare, that all our textbooks were full of 'sophistry and illusion'—colourful condemnation, which, unsurprisingly, didn't go down well with his fellow thinkers, neither then, nor today.

Hume had exaggerated. He derided knowledge excessively—but the seed had been planted, and in time it grew. Thus, when I was learning my philosophical trade in 1958, it continued to rumble on in the background, kept there by 'orthodox' scientists, who desperately hoped that by ignoring it, it would eventually go away. But it didn't. It couldn't. And to crown it all, suddenly, out of the blue, *science* itself proved it to be *true*. At least, in essence.

Following unprecedented success in the late 1800s, by 1900 science was especially pleased with itself. Chemicals, to everyone's surprise, had demonstrated a hidden order and pattern, which seemed to allow them all to fall into their allotted place — it was called the Periodic Table. This appeared to show that all their diverse properties were explicable — they recurred in a predictable, regular pattern. And then, horror of horror, in the 1920s along came the *uncertainty principle*. The electron, which had done so much to establish the regularities in the Periodic Table, declined to join in — it insisted on remaining elusive. Nothing you could do would pin it down. And since nothing moved without electrons — the Periodic Table, especially, made no sense without them — this was a major blow. Of course, like all things 'scientific', you could carry on as if it hadn't happened — *theoretical physicists* in particular clung to 'probabilities', as if that sufficed. It might do in theory. It certainly doesn't in emotional reality. Try — 'The gun is probably not loaded' — 'The atomic weapon is probably safe'. You might accept 'probabilities' as the best we can do — but I don't.

Emotional probability is far too lax for my taste. Human beings can be remarkably *certain* when they try — so how does this work, and where does it come from? What escaped Descartes was the way life coped with *uncertainty* — but that's for later. Here, let's try something that not many scientists do — a bit of 'emotional mathematics'. This book tries out new approaches, so let's see where this one takes us.

We all assume that 2 + 2 = 4 is right. Certainly, it feels that way. And, equally, that 2 + 2 = 5 feels 'wrong'. Note how I slipped a subjective 'feel' into what is perhaps the most basic science of them all — mathematics. I won't ask you what you mean by 'feels right' or 'feels wrong' — we'd be here all day, and still not much the wiser. But I would ask you to note that you did agree with the opening sentences in this paragraph. You agreed that you felt the one was right, and the other wrong. You 'felt'. Is that an emotion?

Assuming that 'feeling' refers essentially to an emotion — what's next? Well in this book, as I'm happy to repeat, we base all on health — healthier acts, thoughts, emotions are preferred to their opposites. There is a scale of goodness, if you like — it's one based on whatever is healthier. Some, like Alec, disagree, at least at first—but I contend that even they are open to persuasion, provided you can build a bridge of *trust*. Because once you do, then, surprise, surprise, you find that they *consent*. They consent, as Alec eventually did, to press for a healthier world—a world we can all agree on, one which you, I, he, she, and all, can accept as basic, as healthier than any other, hence the maxim—no-one-is-safe-until-we're-all-safe.

So, we return to 'I consent, therefore I am'. It might seem to stretch things to add a rider that the *consent* in question refers to accepting health as our number one goal. I need to take a firmer grip of this thread, and persuade it back to the main theme of this book, i.e. war. To fit Descartes's aphorism to this more idealistic objective, we need to change not only the verb, but the pronoun. Thus, we need to replace his original with—'We consent therefore we are healthier'.

I wouldn't want you to consent to something without your full hearted understanding and approval. I asked no less of Lenny, or indeed Alec. What this book aims to do is to secure first your understanding, and then your consent (at a suitably later date) to the higher aphorism—'No-one-is-sane-until-we're-all-sane'.

Nor, as just noted, can we consent to something which clogs the input channel—it takes time and experience to get through. However, the view from the summit is worth the climb—at least it is from my viewpoint. What we're aiming for is to award every human being anywhere, and at any time, the same feeling of existence, or being—'I consent to be alive, therefore I am'. This holds wonderful implications, including delight, music, art and above all peace. At least it does in this book, as the following chapters set out to explore.

The Parental Dilemma

A DILEMMA IS WHERE YOU ARE DAMNED if you do, and damned if you don't—or is that 'jeopardy'? When I think of the *parental dilemma,* these two, and more, overlap. Different readers will attach different meanings to the one, or to the other. And, to crown it all, this 'meaning' will vary from time-to-time, from experience-to-experience. What made perfect sense one time, can seem utterly ridiculous the next—and vice-versa—even within the same person. Which is awkward, when all the time you are trying to remain heathy, to stay alive as healthily as possible—at least that's what it's safest to assume.

What follows from this is that you need constantly to check the validity of the source. Has the info from that person proved reliable in the past? Or are they trying to sell you a line? See how easily that slips into — can you *trust* them? Are they telling you the *truth?* And, ultimately, do you *consent* to proceed on the basis that they are doing both of these? *Truth, trust* and *consent* — the Triple Values — I did find them so useful in Parkhurst Prison — pragmatism, that's the key. What works, as opposed to what you think works. Or, to stretch things a little further — to what's real.

And having emphasised just how helpless the toddler is, how dependent on the reliability of those so much bigger than him or her (or you) at the time, we need now to reverse roles. From looking at things from the toddler's point of view, we change to that of the parent. Being helpless can be so painful, it pays you to 'forget' it as soon as you can — so the toddler-view certainly did need emphasising in this book, since too many remain stuck there, and need extra help to escape their *nursery nightmares.* But why do they? What needs to happen for you to progress, to leave emotional dependency behind, and stand on your own two feet emotionally? Well, in a word, education — emotional education at that. Asking your consent. Persuading you to think for yourself. Giving you options. Genuine options — do you want to play with the bricks, or not? It is easy to forget that human beings remember. They carry things over from one scenario to the next, and sometimes they don't notice how much has changed — in a word, they fail to adapt.

And one of the biggest changes is to go from infant to parent. Suddenly you have this squawking creature who needs you, in order to stay alive. They can take zero responsibility for themselves — why, they can't even turn over in bed by themselves — so unless you keep them alive, they're dead. Heavy? I should say so. And if you're not too comfortable with doing the right thing for yourself, to keep you alive — here's an extra burden you have to cope with on top of all the rest. And quite an insistent burden that can be. 'Waaaaah' comes all too close. A dilemma — I should say.

Let's move this on a couple of years to when toddling begins. You watch as your young charge takes her or his first tentative steps. If you're nice and confident yourself, then you'll find it easy to be encouraging — 'Yes, you can do it. I did it. It's not easy to begin with — but you're a capable lass/lad, so you'll soon pick it up — like I did'.

But suppose your confidence level is not very high. Lenny's wasn't. So when your little girl or little boy starts tottering, you rush in to prevent worse. All you have to do is keep a tight hold of their hand, and that'll stop them falling over and cracking their skull on the curb. Sounds simple. You are big and strong enough to prevent them falling to their doom. You're in charge. You're the adult-in-the-room. You are the one with the responsibility. If you don't ensure they remain upright, any damage that happens to them is laid firmly at your door. Move, or they're dead.

And of course, that's perfectly real, perfectly proper. If you don't look after your offspring, who will? They can't—they're far too small, too weak, too incapable. No, being a parent places heavy responsibilities on your shoulders. And of course, to begin with, it's incredibly easy. All you have to do is to pick them up, put them where you know it's safe, and make sure they remain so. And yet. That's not all. Something missing here. You're in charge now—but for how long?

What happens is they grow bigger. They start small, we all do. But then they put on height. They grow out of their clothes, and start moving under their own steam. What are you going to do? When you're fully in control you can ensure nothing untoward happens to them—they're safe, they feel comfortable, and so do you. But then they start making moves to go beyond—to reach out for themselves, where your writ doesn't run. The feet they are standing on are their own. Or are they?

Here's the dilemma. When do you loose go? How soon do you give them more leeway? The longer you are fully in charge, the longer you can assure yourself, and them, that you can limit any damage that might lurk. But, and it's a big but—hang on too long and they'll never learn to walk for themselves. Walking is not easy, as any toddler will confirm for you. But never progressing from crawling to bipedal can be worse, far worse.

And just as you can never tell precisely where an electron is, while at the same time measuring where it is going—so the *parental dilemma* hits not one or two parents, but every single one, including, Dear Reader, your good self, if you are, or have been one. Nor is there a simple, single, or *universal* answer—people vary, toddlers vary—and unless you keep up with that, with the wishes, decisions, and yes, *consents*, of your offspring, then you'll be out of sync, and will not be performing optimally. It's the same with educators the world over. Go too fast, and you overload the mind's input channel. Go too slow, and your 'pupils' are bored. So how to keep to the happy middle way? How to judge if you're doing it optimally. Well, my answer, as it is to all apparently intractable human problems, is 'together'. No-one-is-safe-until-we're-all-safe.

'IT TAKES A VILLAGE TO BRING UP A CHILD'—this is a wonderfully apt saying, and at its heart is the *parental dilemma*. Ask what other parents are doing. Learn from their mistakes. Gain comfort and security from sharing your challenge—oh, and by the way, your offspring will enjoy playing with theirs—provided you can rinse out the bullying.

Ah yes—bullies. Sadly, toddlers aren't the only ones who bully. Some keep it up all their adult lives too. They forget the difference between infancy and adulthood. They keep thinking that if they hit people that'll help. If they frighten others, then that will somehow promote them. It doesn't. The world around us, our environment, our reality, trundles on whether we like it or not—the only way to survive in it, that is to say to remain in the least bit healthy, is to find out as much as you can about what is happening out there. We none of us have eyes in the back of our head—we, every one of us, need input from all around, to keep our data on reality as up-to-date and as comprehensive as we can.

Blindspots are the very devil. And bullying breeds them like there's no tomorrow. It's simple enough really, if you can think straight about it. Don't cut yourself off from vital sources of data. Worse—it sounds so easy—don't punch them into shape, make sure they take your line, knock out any 'free-thinkers', 'dissenters', all those who decline to think you are 'The Greatest'. As a parent, or a demagogue, you certainly have the power. But have a care. The shape you knock them into would have to be your shape, that'd be the 'gain' from your position. But look at what you're losing. Strange as it may sound, you could actually benefit from their viewpoint. Their take on this endlessly complicated world of ours could make all the difference. The very fact that they take a different view to your own could help. All right you do get kooks out there—you do need to sort the wheat from the chaff—but 'twas ever thus. And the odd tyrant or global bully isn't going to change that, just because they want to.

And health turns on *consent,* especially mental health. Consent is to agree freely, because you want to, not because you've been bullied into it. Consent means you've been given the chance to evaluate all the alternatives, all the options, and have drawn your own conclusion, and have freely, voluntarily, and willingly consented. Quite a cocktail, and not always easy to obtain, or ensure. But, if you want to share views of reality—and that's the only possible way through—then you need to stop all bullying, eradicate it wherever you can, and listen. 'Listen to the patient, she or he's telling you the diagnosis' said William Osler. And by diagnosis he meant reality—in his case, the reality behind the disease you've been asked to assist with—but I expand this to include all reality. If trustworthy people tell you it's safe to proceed, then that increases your confidence to do so. But if your sources of info have been bullied, have been coerced, and are therefore giving you not what they really see, but what they've been taught to say—then you, they, and with war all of us, are in trouble. Bullies need identifying, and eliminating—and to do this, we need lots of adults-in-the-room. Bring them on. Because doing so can be delightful.

Consensual Delights

DO YOU HAVE AGENCY? By which I do *not* mean are you an estate agent, a special agent, or running an employment agency. No, this refers to you acting as an agent *for yourself*. Just pause for a moment, and ask what do these other 'agents' do? Well, they each do their own thing. If you want to sell a house, steal your competitor's secrets, find yourself a job, then you do the best you can yourself, and when you need something extra you call in help. You don't think twice about it—sell your house yourself if you can, no question—but if it doesn't go, then call in assistance. Nothing wrong with that. Nothing to be ashamed of. You balance up the factors available to you, you then decide, or, to put it another way, you then *consent* to follow the best plan available to you. It's all a matter of course, it all goes through without question—it may have hiccoughs along the way, and if it's complicated, as it often is, it may take longer. But you know what these other agents do—so what about yourself? How much do you know about what *you* do?

As before, I like to find rules-of-thumb which apply to one and all. I take delight in uncovering items, or 'facts' which don't just apply to me, but universally, preferably to every single human being ever born. This isn't such an odd endeavour—it's something which everyone does, once in a while—and so it is itself just such a universal human 'trend'. Now the central theme of this book is health — that's to say, living life to the full, enjoying being well, rather than being ill. And when considering consensual delights, it helps to go back to medical basics.

Take breathing for example. It's something we all do. Once we stop, then we stop altogether. No need to dwell on the negative, though it does play a major part in a doctor's workload — you have four minutes to decide if the patient in front of you is still breathing — after that, other considerations are of lesser import. I didn't make this up. This is a central fact of life. Breathe, or you are done for.

Let's take a leaf out of a scientist's book and set out to define breathing. Well, you open your mouth, and suck in air. That doesn't cover it all. Sometimes you breathe in through your nose. Why the difference? Once you start getting pernickety about the details, you can spend a lifetime working them all out, and still miss the main point. You breathe to keep yourself alive. It may seem obvious, but that doesn't mean it doesn't need pointing out.

And here's where agency matters. You do your own breathing. No-one can breathe for you. You're the one who burns the oxygen you breathe in, and it's your carbon dioxide you breathe out. No-one else's. Why labour the point? Well, because some childhoods rob you, they leave you bereft in the agency department, they emphasise what you can't do, not what you can. In this book I set out to reverse that trend. You do your own breathing. You do your own thinking. You do your own agency. You do your own creativity.

See how I slipped that in? 'Art' is so often for other people. 'I don't know much about art, but I know what I like' — this, too often, is used as a put down, a disparagement. It implies that others are cleverer than you, they know more, so they seem superior. But don't forget, they don't breathe for you. And, in this context, they don't do delight, for you. That's something you do for yourself, something only you can do.

So where does delight come from? Again, it's all too easy to get lost in words. But words point to a more concrete reality — they refer to something bigger. In this case to breathing in-and-out. Which, if you let it, can be delightful. Fill your lungs on a brisk spring morning, or when looking out to sea — what a delightful experience that can be, if you let it. This gives weight to the point that delight is as intrinsic to being alive as breathing is. It's your birthright. It's what you do. Simply being alive means taking in oxygen, and taking in fresh air can be delightful.

Of course, breathing can become so everyday, it ceases to signify. You get on with the rest of your life, without being overly concerned as to where your next breath is coming from. But it's there, it's always there, until it's not. It's the same with delight. It's waiting round every corner, it's part and parcel of being alive—you may need to learn, you may need some training, especially some emotional education—but it's what you do, or what you can do. It's built into your very own agency. Find something you can add to, something where what you do makes a difference—and that's where delight is to be found. Fresh ideas, like fresh air are available to all, all who are healthy that is.

Before we leave breathing, let's bring mouth-to-mouth into the discussion. If you find someone who is nearly drowning, you can bring them back to life by covering their mouth with yours, and blowing your stale air into their lungs. You are actually breathing for them. It's a joint effort. You are adding to their oxygen intake, when they can't do it for themselves. You can't keep it up indefinitely, but your contribution can be lifesaving. In effect, you are sharing your life-giving breath. Not to be sniffed at. In fact, when you think about it, it's quite remarkable. Sharing saves lives. Now that's another of those universal facts about human beings, and a rather delightful one too.

Widen this to the rest of life, and you find that participating in how others have solved life's ever-changing problems helps. Not only helps, but when conditions are propitious, is a source of delight, indeed a reliable, constant source. People's tastes, their experiences, their 'likes' differ—but what is always the same, is the fact that life throws up problems, and living organisms, such as ourselves, solve them. Watching, joining in, breathing with—all these add significantly to consensual delights. Even the wide range of delightfulness adds to the beauty of it. Some prefer one avenue, others different paths—but what they are all doing is joining in joint ventures. Socialising can be delightful. It can also be problematic, and lead to destructions, as we've noted—but the more fruitful message, the healthier view is that human beings enjoy being delighted. They enjoy socialising. Whenever they can, they find it delightful. You don't have to be special, but you do have to be awake.

Sex is oversold. Medically speaking, its function is to fertilise, so ensuring we don't die out. But the two humans involved are not always emotionally healthy, hazards which sex tends to gloss over, while doing nothing to address them. From my years as a family doctor, sex is perhaps best seen as a conversation — if you're on speaking terms, it's more likely to go well. But either way, the sex bit is essentially transient — it doesn't last. Nor does the 'auto-pilot' element, which offers a by-pass to having to think. Worse, in rather too many contexts, sex can be weaponised — so confusing sex with 'love' can be entirely counterproductive.

But to return to the subject of 'agency', do you view yourself as an actor, a doer, someone who, in however small a way, makes a difference? Or, sadly, have you, like Lenny (Line 263) been 'brainwashed into fear'? This is where placing 'health' centre stage adds so much to the mix — very simple, very straightforward, quite independent of who or where you (or I) come from — we all prefer being well to being ill. And the real advantage of the former is that it offers a sure-fire avenue to delight — at least it does in my book. Which, again, is why war robs us all of so much. And before being delighted, we need to return to the clinic, and see where war does come from, and what, if any, remedies we can find for it. To this we now turn.

CHAPTER 6

Is War Disease Curable?

Guff-disease— Where's an Adult-in-the-Room When You Need
One?— Prevention is Better Than Cure—Dynamic Security

Guff-disease

AS A SELF-APPOINTED GLOBAL DOCTOR, I have had to make one or two assumptions. In the normal course of medical practice, a patient comes to see you with a problem—something is causing them trouble, else they wouldn't bother coming. This carries with it both spoken, and unspoken conditions. First, do no harm—whatever I do mustn't make things worse than they already are. Thus nothing I write here impugns the courage, determination or fortitude of the military. They do things which most of us would quail from, and indeed would run a mile from doing.

Courage and imagination in soldiers have been rightly admired over the ages. I wouldn't want to change that, nor indeed challenge it. Had my father and so many others not gone to war in 1939, Hitler would undoubtedly have destroyed more, far more, than he actually did. As a doctor, especially one who worked with murderers, I need to operate in a neutral fashion—accepting those social norms which help understand the disease, while entertaining novel techniques which penetrate to its roots, and thereafter to its cure, especially when it is widely assumed there isn't one.

So just as nothing I said or did condoned murder, I would never subtract from the bravery of those who take up arms to protect us all. When a disease is well advanced, radical and potentially destructive surgery is the only course available. I'm thinking of some forms of cancer, such as melanoma, when the whole leg needs amputating, to stop the disease spreading further. Radical, drastic, most regrettable—but, by the time the disease is already too well-established, there is little else available for us to do. So it is with war. Once it's destructivity is well advanced, and all efforts at prevention have failed—what else can you do? The question I put, and indeed ask every reader to face up to, is—'Is that really the best we can do?' Wait for the next one, and then smash whatever needs smashing? Far better to explore alternatives, while there is still time. In the case of melanoma, screen through the multiple causative factors, and cut out those you can (especially sunbathing). I ask nothing more with war—it is a disease, it has many threads, it can be most confusing—but none of this should stop us thinking, stop us wondering if there isn't a better way—and then insisting on implementing it. Plan B is never more urgently needed.

The thing I do emphasise about war is—what a waste. All this splendid valour, intelligence, even creativity is expended—on what? In a word, on *guff*. Just as the current Supreme Court of the United States cannot sensibly account for why it sanctions killing people—so murderers, and especially warmongers, make no sense when asked why. Which is what this book is all about. There is a reason, as there was for every murderer I examined—but (as already discussed at some length) the perpetrator cannot tell you, or themselves, what that reason is. Indeed, the whole thrust of this book is that when they can—it goes.

Guff needs emphasising. Agatha Christie, and most of Hollywood keep peddling the myth that murderers, and by implication warmongers, know what they're doing. They don't. The reasons they don't go way back into the past. And, if you try and follow them too abruptly, then it can be the worse for you—as I found with Alec and his garrotte, and as innumerable enquirers (so-called free thinkers) find when they prod demagogues too precisely. Don't expose their vulnerability, else they'll defend themselves against you in a most aggressive manner. Yet unless their impotence is exposed, then it will continue indefinitely, and can only get progressively worse, as it always does. Putin escalates for just the same reasons Hitler did—they are (or were) trying to solve their unseen problem, using powerful but self-defeating reasoning to do so.

What if my explanation that friendless childhoods breed warring adults is *true*? What then? Well, this immediately shines a blistering light on the whole topic. We can see, examine, and improve childhoods for free, indeed for profit—their very own adult taxes pay for the input, as described. But above all, we can understand. We can deploy our ineffable thinking facilities in an open, transparent way. It all makes sense, gruesome of course, but hold your nose, and look.

Toddlers squabble—does that really need scientific scrutiny? Can't we accept that as read? Any who need convincing should visit a badly run kindergarten, and watch. Don't interfere, and you can see for yourself that unhappy toddlers hit, bully, abuse and try to dominate any other toddler within reach. It happens at the drop of a hat. It's not unusual. It's not insane. It is so 'normal' that some observers give up and assume it's genetic—which it isn't.

All that needs to happen for toddler squabbling to transfer, unimproved, onto the battlefield, or into the trenches, is to show that fear blocks thought. And quite remarkably, along come unimpeachable scientific brain scans to prove precisely this. And, wow, do they prove it? They do so without introspection, but with full objectivity, repeatability, and the obviousness of any scientific device—why this ultra-scientific evidence, unique in all psychiatry, still fails to penetrate so many psychiatrists' doctrines, is scary.

Play an audio tape to a person who has been traumatised. If the tape is benign, their frontal lobes and speech centres continue to function as normal. The brainscan wave patterns confirm this, in a way that is obvious, overt and irrefutable for all who take it upon themselves to look. However, if the audio tape is of the gunshot, or car crash, or whatever it was which terrified that particular sufferer from that particular trauma—then their brain seizes up. They have a 'stroke'. Their frontal lobes stop. Their thinking doesn't work anymore—it's 'muddled'. They are rendered speechless with terror. Which means that their trauma never goes away. It never leaves them. Because they cannot recall it clearly, they are unable to think it through.

They need help, but can't ask for it, because they don't know anything's wrong. This is why it never ceases in their heads. In Alec's case his father was forever throwing his mother down the stairs. For Lenny, his mother continued to batter him, even though he was incarcerated in a maximum-security prison into which even I had difficulty entering, let alone an 80-year-old woman. Sceptics are invited to check out Lenny's video (see *Appendix 1*)—his fear is palpable—but, as clarity improves, so does his cure.

Trauma stops humans thinking. Homo sapiens becomes homo non-sapiens. Bullied toddlers then go on to bully everyone within range. More trauma is inflicted, enmity becomes endemic, and the *guff-disease* proliferates. It's long-lasting and infectious. If you thought Covid was bad—take a look at terror.

Which brings us to the next difference between treating an individual in my clinic and prescribing for a global population. With a person, as I did with Lenny and Alec, I can question them as to where this *guff* comes from. In Lenny's case, why did he continue to fear his mother when he was no longer half her size? And for Alec—his mother didn't die, indeed she was later able to confirm his change of heart in a way that only the blindest could fail to be moved by. The important point is that they *consented*. They gave their consent to listen to my opinion, to tell me all that I needed to know, and thereafter, to give serious consideration to doing what I prescribed. Note there are already large holes in this process, some of which we have already discussed. But *consent* is crucial—persuasion not coercion, or as my favourite Early Quaker, James Nayler, put it, with infinite wisdom—'it takes its kingdom by entreaty, not with contention'. What insight. What clarity. And all of 363 years ago.

Let's try this out on Putin. Try saying—'Now, Vladimir, you don't know what you're doing, so stop until you do. You can't give a sensible explanation for destroying as much of Ukraine as you can get away with—so cease and desist immediately. Guff, that's your problem.'

Look at how he reacts to the brave people who try this. I have in mind that remarkable TV presenter who held up a sign behind the newscaster. What happened to her? I dread to think. Look at all the 'laws' his puppet legislature impose—making even half-sensible criticism of the insanity of his war strictly illegal and subject to arrest and imprisonment, or worse. Once his thinking is blocked, once his frontals are seized up, once he is afflicted with *muddled thought*—then all you can expect from him is ever more *guff*. How can it not be?

And more to the point, how can you doubt that frozen frontals account for his veering ever further from thoughtfulness. Something must account for it. It's not genetic. If you can come up with a better explanation, then do so, only be quick about it. And for confirmation, look at all the other demagogues, or would be demagogues—both in the USA, in the UK, and sadly enough, around the world. When you hear 'I'm the greatest. I need to reign forever and ever and ever and ever. No-one can criticise me. If you sneer at me, I'll crush you'—just try adding—'and by the way, I'm an unmitigated and inveterate toddler', and it all begins to make sense.

Once you can see where the problem is coming from, then, and only then can you begin to think up viable remedies. I claim to have cured serial killers. Not something that conventional wisdom allows for, so the Government of the day crushed it. But it still makes sense, at least it does to me—and, more important, it shines a welcome light on what to do next, to which we now turn.

Where's an Adult-in-the-Room When You Need One?

IF TODDLER-SQUABBLES WRIT LARGE do account for our war disease, what's the remedy? Well, the best route to clarity in such a murky field is to keep things as simple as you can, and go back to square one. How would you stop toddlers squabbling? When one of these obstreperous (and rather larger than you) two-year-olds grabs your favourite toy—what would you do? Well, obviously 'Waaaaah' comes easily to mind. But that doesn't stop it. You, being too small, need external help, just as I did when Alec threatened to kill me. Nothing wrong with asking for help. We are none of us Super(wo)man. We may be tremendous, but we're only human, and we all have our limitations, without exception. Help, from those around, is vital. It only becomes problematic when enmity is endemic and *truth, trust* and *consent* sparse.

The remedy is the adult-in-the-room. You are too small, or you don't have the authority, or the muscle—so you import these necessary ingredients from someone who does. This is obvious enough in kindergartens. Those in charge are known to have the required status and authority. They are paid to look after their charges. They develop their own way of responding. They find out which approaches work best, and when they are consistent apply these without fear or favour.

Transfer this on to the wider society and though the answer may not be as clear cut, it is just as necessary. *Toddler-thinking* occurs all too often, and every society takes measures to limit it, not all of which are cost-effective. We need to note very carefully what works on the smallest scale, before seeing if we can extrapolate it across the globe. Every sensible kindergarten has a naughty corner, or equivalent. Toddlers need to learn to cooperate. Some do so without demur. Others have hidden agendas, their families of origin leave much to be desired, so they throw their weight about whenever they get the chance. Only badly run kindergartens tolerate this.

So how do you stop anti-social behaviour in two-year-olds? Well, what do they understand? It is crucial to enlist their thinking, their reasoning, even pre-verbal. They may not be able to say the words 'naughty corner', but it is your job, as a kindergarten teacher, to ensure they know what it is, and at least as important, what it is for. But, whatever you do, don't overdo it. When Alec was put in the block (meaning in solitary confinement), the last thing I wanted to happen was that he learnt anew that he was impotent, he could do nothing to improve things—his nascent agency was shot. I wanted to ensure that he knew that any action taken against him was commensurate, that it was fair, and that it didn't rule out his being able to resume speaking to me in the future. Precisely the same happens to two-year-olds. They can reason, just as Ethan could on arrival. And since our objective is that *they* do the controlling of their un-socialisms, from the inside, then it is quite essential that nothing we do curtails this, in the least degree.

'You hit Tommy, so we'll hit you.' What does that teach the growing mind? It teaches it that the bigger and stronger you are, then you can do what you like. That, in the old phrase, brawn matters more than brain. And, since we're looking to understand warring adults, it teaches them to get ever bigger and ever mightier weapons, so they can easily 'win' any argument, whether over territory, such as the Ukraine, or whatever. Might is *right*, as Bismarck had it, and possession is 9/10 of the law. Absolutely correct for badly run kindergartens. But also a clear recipe for World Wars—One, Two, and here's desperately hoping, not Three.

You reason with them. Yes, you talk to them. You translate your meanings into words and gestures they can follow. You smile, you encourage them to think. You are friendly, so that they learn that that's what adults are for. And you explain, in language they can understand, that if they do hit Tommy again, then they will automatically have to spend time out of the social group. The social contract is not negotiable. If you want to be sociable, if you want to stay in, be aware that that requires you to desist from being anti-social. If you deviate from this, you're out. Put it more positively—social delight defeats social harm. The norm, the healthy situation is that human beings of any age prefer social contact to social isolation. Even Ethan did, and he'd only been here a couple of minutes.

Did you notice I slipped in — 'That's what adults are for'? Kindergartens, especially those inspired by Head-Start, or Sure-Start, set out to teach their clients a lesson — at least the most fruitful ones do. And what are their objectives? What is it that they need to teach most? Well, we discussed teaching them choices, options, learning that you giving, or withholding *consent* makes all the difference. Why is this important? Well, though you may not have any control over whether that bigger toddler runs off with your invaluable dolly — you need to learn, indeed you need to be taught that this is not optimal. The best way to survive in this challenging world is to learn that there are bits of it you *can* control. If you put your mind to it, you can cope.

This may seem so obvious it doesn't need repeating. But the world is full of people who have never been taught it — they have never learnt that they really do have agency, and that this can make all the difference. In this book, it makes the difference between health and unhealth. And in the ultimate, between peace and war. If you've never been shown that what you do can impact, what you struggle with can in fact improve matters — then how can you ever know?

Look at some recent (and on-going) politicians. They lie. Why? Well in this book the answer is *nursery nightmares*. They are frozen in a kindergarten world where, whatever they do, they cannot stop bigger, more obstreperous people snatching what's most precious from them. They have never been taught that they have an element of control. Nothing like Super(wo)man — but enough to get by, if exercised judiciously. It sounds complicated — it isn't. It sounds like a fairytale — which is what it will always remain for those whose toddlerhood never showed them anything else. Do you matter? When were you taught this? If you don't count, can you believe where your self-doubt started? And if you can, are you prepared to undergo re-training to correct it?

Vladimir Putin lies. Donald Trump lies. Boris Johnson lies. Lying comes as naturally as breathing. And this is where it all starts — if you've no control, no agency over what happens to you. As a toddler (all toddlers) your immediate future is not, by definition, in your hands. You are fed and watered by others, else you're not. You need to learn to take ever-increasing responsibility for yourself, for your own actions, your own agency, your own food and drink, your own survival. Your future needs placing in your very own hands, just as the two feet you learn to walk about on are your own.

When in this book we look for explanations as to why this healthy transition doesn't happen, we need only look at childhoods. Kindergartens are fun, if you're cherished. They're hell, if you're not. And for some, they remain an ongoing nightmare, in which the future is as bleak as the past, and just as immutable. Without agency, without choice, without being asked for your *consent*—then nothing changes. Your *nursery nightmare* continues, willy-nilly. It didn't stop when you were small, so why should it stop now? *Toddler thinkers* have little interest in the present, and less in the future. Why bother, when it's not your responsibility and there's nothing you can do about it? Worse, without *nutritious emotions*, life is bleak, and will forever remain so. You try all sorts of drastic remedies, Hitler tried invading Poland—but nothing hits the spot, because it's the wrong spot. *Nutritious emotions* are not to be found by crushing people.

What do we do now? Well, first we need clarity. Next, we need to find the wider equivalent of the naughty corner—something everyone understands, and accepts. We could start by making it illegal to lie about public policy. We already do this for commerce—you can't sell a product on a fairytale prospectus. In New Zealand, it's illegal to lie in politics—something we should all legislate for across the world, if we're interested in global health.

Next, we need to establish adults-in-the-room. When things are going toddler-shaped, we need people we can refer to, who we can call on for help. Reliable, helpful, trustworthy adult-type people. We already have some on a local scale—police, courts, responsible media and press—though not enough. Nicaragua shows what can be done. We need more. Indeed, we need every participant in every society to take as much responsibility as falls their way to resist, to withdraw their *consent*, to agitate for an end to *toddler-thinking*. A big ask? It certainly is. But *nursery nightmares* are hellish, and if you can curtail them, then we (and they) will all benefit—we might even survive that bit longer too.

Prevention is Better Than Cure

WE NEED UNIMPUGNABLE adults-in-the-room. This is not easy to achieve. We need police, army and judiciary we can trust—again *trust* is something that must be earned. It's fragile, and can easily be lost, and corrupted, especially by liars. But there are ways of building it. There are ways of measuring it. But it's something that needs everyone to take a hand in. Wherever you see standards slipping, you need to say so. Wherever deceit is being practised, you need to whistleblow. And if you hear of whistleblowing, then help it along, don't hinder it. It might be painful, especially if it involves re-thinking — but add your thinking to the mix. You matter too.

I like to think of us all as belonging to a single living organism — one composed of hundreds, millions, even billions of other human beings, each one of which is more like us than not. It's how living organisms work. You yourself are composed of trillions of separate cells. Indeed 600 million years ago, life forms worked out how to change from the single-celled versions that was all there was before, to multi-cellular monsters. In my understanding, this came about through the construction of a particular chemical that had never been there before — it goes by the acronym DHA, and we get ours from fish, who, in turn, get theirs from even smaller sea creatures that live in the plankton. It's a fascinating omega-6 fatty acid. Our brains consist of it more than of anything else. It has a curious way with electrons — in fact, some have called it *nature's* semi-conductor. But this is a topic for later.

We are each individuals with our own brains, our own minds, and our own two legs — or we should be. And just as the leg muscles need to coordinate with everything else, if we are ever to put one foot in front of another — so too, at a social, indeed global level, every single human needs to coordinate their agencies towards a healthier whole. This means correcting all deviations from adult reality that we see. Comment on it, make a fuss about it, move, so that it becomes less. Every single cell in your body does nothing less. They all work together in remarkable harmony. It's only when one or two branch out on their own, and you get something equivalent of cellular anarchy, otherwise known as cancer.

This book is based on health, it sets out to promote it, it seeks out disease, especially among those who promote social ill health. So here we can recall that ancient Chinese precept about the three types of doctor. The ordinary doctor treats disease — that's something we are all familiar with, especially when ill. The middling doctor prevents disease — a laudable calling, if you can persuade enough people to follow your prescriptions. But, so the aphorism runs, the best doctor prevents war. Now this is not so commonplace. And of course, as with all preventive measures, the doctor can prescribe, but unless others in society take notice, little is achieved. Persuasion is key. And before you or I would *consent,* we need to be clear, we need to see which bit goes where, and how our individual contribution can add to the general overall weal, or health.

So let's review the *triple values,* and see how each contributes to preventing war. First we have *truth.* Is it true that war is founded *on guff?* If you remove the guff, does war go? Is this reasonable? Does it work? The difficulty here is that if you ask warmongers directly, they obfuscate—just like murderers do. Why did you kill her/him? 'S/he had it coming.' 'A red mist came down.' 'I just lost it.' Nothing you can get your teeth into. It's the same with warmongers, and other *toddler thinkers.* 'Ukraine has always been part of Mother Russia.' 'Sovereignty matters most.' 'We need to remember history, and get back to Greatness.' 'We're revenging the wrongs that your forefathers did to us.'

When you look closely at these, they don't ring *true.* Of course, they are emotive, they wow lots of people—everyone likes to be the *greatest,* especially those who never felt this, when they were too small to do it for themselves. But emotions can cloud the issue—clarity is difficult to maintain when feelings run riot. But there is a reality out there, waiting to see if we make a hash of it—and boiling us to a frazzle, if we miss.

We need to be as accurate in our statements as we possibly can be. *Truth,* in this book, is the degree to which our mental world reflects the real world. It can never be 100%—we keep hoping it will be, and some think *science* can take us there. But the reality is our human faculties are limited. We get things wrong. And if they are too wrong, we become first ill, then dead. If our media propagate untruths, people suffer and then die. Just because *truth* is never *absolute* doesn't mean it doesn't matter. The fact that it is always partial means we need constantly to shore it up, we need to do our best to ensure it is as accurate, as precise as possible. We'll never get perfection—but we can have fun getting there.

So to *trust.* Trust is relying on another's *truth.* Truth can never be 100%—it is simply the degree to which what you think is out there really is. Trust is how much credence you give to what other people tell you. If you're sensible, you divide people into groups, some more trustworthy, others less. And it matters. It matters for health. Suppose I tell you there is enough oxygen in this room for both of us—do you trust me? If you do, and there is, then we're both fine. If you don't, and I'm wrong, we both suffer. I can't know everything, nor can you—I rely on what I'm told, just as you do—and *trust* in this context impacts directly on health. Not only yours and mine, but globally. Without *trust*, war looms.

Trust needs earning. You can build it up incrementally—small things make all the difference. Pay attention to detail. Be meticulous. Exercise your 'intent' to ensure that you say and do things which improve health and creativity, rather than not. Again, so much depends on what you picked up from your childhood. If you were shown that trusting people was beneficial all round, then you would try it out for yourself and find that you could make vastly more progress with it than without.

However, if you had to rely on make-believe, on the notion that since *nutritious emotions* were scarce, if you wanted them, which we all do, you had to invent them—then your 'truths' would be based on pretends, not on the reality we share. Our realities would differ, and, following this, so would our health.

As far as I'm concerned, I don't want you to accept what I say as the truth. Don't take my word for it. Find out if it makes sense, if it applies to the world around you. If it does, act on it. If it doesn't, modify it so that it does. My responsibility is limited. I needed to work out as best I could what made most sense to me—which happily I did. Having done that to my satisfaction (and delight), I next needed to express it, write about it, communicate it as clearly as I possibly could. Again, this is never 100%, I'm no Shakespeare, and even he muddles things from time-to-time. Read it, puzzle over it, and if it makes sense, do something about it.

So, to the third leg of the peace-of-mind—*consent*. This really is the glue that holds the other two together. Peace-of-mind is not possible without a good dollop of these *three values*. But you also have to see the sense in them, they have to make sense to you, you have to make them your own—only then can they prove to be worthwhile.

Now I'm not going to *consent* to something that makes no sense to me. Guff is outside my comfort zone. But, and this is where it bites—until such as Putin *consent* to the fact that they are acting on *guff*, that their very purpose in life is out of sync, then our peace-of-mind is at sea, and the peace of the world, at risk. This book, naturally, says such aggressors need bringing up to date—they need to re-synchronise their emotions, so that they diminish the guff, and replace it with more fruitful cogitations.

It's hard to know how to do this. It took two years constant and very careful work with such as Alec. And even then, he reverted at one point, and added me to his hit list. But see how we won through in the end. He did *consent* to discuss his terrors. He did agree that he had been unable to think straight. And, even more important, he saw the value in doing so. Admittedly such as Putin, and others, pose a bigger challenge to our way through—how you persuade them to reverse their plottings, and *consent* to a healthier behaviour, is not an easy one to solve. But, so far, we have not even begun—and until we do, then Nucleargeddon looms.

Just listen to what Alec had to say, when, later, he was able to think more clearly. He confidently told me that if you have a tantrum when you're four, then you stamp your foot on the ground. But have one when you're 24, and some-one dies. Or someone invades Ukraine. No easier to deal with than advanced melanoma—but for pity's sake, let's start.

Dynamic Security

CAN OUR WAR-DISEASE BE PREVENTED? Well, obviously not until we know where it comes from. Scurvy killed many a long-distance mariner, until its origins in lack of vitamin C became not only known, but implemented. Nowadays, you can travel to the moon without your teeth falling out simply because you didn't eat the right food. But it took the Royal Navy half a century before this known fact of human health became obligatory. We simply don't have the time for that today.

Apparently, the Royal Navy took so long because they feared being accused of incompetence. Men died at sea because their commanders had failed them. True, in one sense—but the failure initially derived from ignorance. Are we destined to die too, because our commanders don't want to appear weak, or unknowing? Or do they genuinely not know that toddlers will squabble, whereas adults socialise? And if they don't know—who is going to tell them? If we live in a real democracy—government by the people—then it's the people who need to speak up—and since we are the people, that means you and me—once we *consent*.

On the assumption that war, murder, and indeed violence in general comes from within, and not from without—how can it best be prevented? Well, an adult-in-the-room is a prerequisite. But how should they intervene? Too heavy handed, and they'll guarantee to make things worse. Too ineffectual, and they might as well not bother—they'd be no help to you.

Let's go to a situation where violent challenges are faced routinely—prison. Prisoners take hostages, they plot dastardly revenge, including death. In recent correspondence with Charlie Bronson, one of the UK's most notorious, and most misinterpreted prisoners,[4] he tells me he has taken eleven hostages, including three prison governors, a doctor, and even his own lawyer. So, you're on duty when the call comes through to you—Bronson has done it again, he's taken yet another hostage—what are you going to do about it?

Well, you could call in the sharp shooters, as one of the prisoners on C-Wing told me they did to him. Or you could negotiate. If, like the Royal Navy, you deemed this to be beneath you, then your intervention would make things worse. Prisoners are violent, so let's be more violent back—doesn't make sense, and it doesn't work. It's the opposite of what I did when I went to C-Wing in the first place. I did not arm myself up to the teeth, put on a bullet proof vest, or a garrotte-proof collar. No, I set out with a clear goal—murder came from the past, and I needed to find out when, why, and how best to put it right. Happily, the Government's Minister in charge didn't tumble to what I was doing for a while, so let me do it for five years unencumbered. Pity it wasn't longer, but *muddled thinking* prevails.

Would my approach work in prisons more widely? This is exactly the sort of conversation I had had with the prison officer I've called Colin earlier in this book. He was the one who shepherded Alec into C-Wing in the first place. Had he not been in charge in Reception that day, Alec would have insisted on going down to the block, or come onto the wing determined to do enough to get himself off it. And being resolute, his withdrawal of *consent* to remain on C-Wing, his determination would have prevailed—neither I, nor anyone else, would have had a chance.

---

4. Also nowadays known as Charles Salvador.

But Colin reversed the standard prison approach, and appealed to Alec's reason. Alec sensed that something inside was wrong, but he didn't know what — the last thing on his mind was his father's violence, and he was determined to keep it that way. But because Colin treated him like a reasoning person, Alec responded, and agreed to come. It took some two years to grow him up emotionally — but happily, with him at least, we had the time.

You are called to the scene — Bronson, as usual, is backing his complaints with violence — you have to act fast — but what? Use force, as Bronson is doing, and you too may smash things. Find someone who can talk to Bronson, and he or she might be able to talk him down, instead of taking him down. Because I can tell you from direct personal knowledge there is a reason Bronson took his hostages — even a doctor and his lawyer — hardly rational. No, what lay behind Bronson's act is a grievance. If he could have found a channel of communication he could trust, believe me, he would not have done it. But he couldn't, so he did.

What he needed, ever since I examined him on Friday morning, 5 July 1991 (the first of several), was to be listened to. He needed, as the phrase has it, 'a good listening to'. In common with all lawbreakers, he felt he had been wronged, and his violent actions were his inept way of putting that right. It didn't work. It got worse. No-one in the prison system spent the time talking him down. I prepared quite a number of medico-legal reports for him — two of which he even re-printed verbatim in one of his books[5] — but time and opportunity to unpack his inner tensions were never afforded either of us.

And what was the gist of my talks with Colin? We discussed hostage-taking. We talked about the standard, unthinking prison approach. And we agreed on the main principles of what should better be done, as his later conversation with Alec showed. Standard prison protocol is called 'locks, bolts and bars'. It's self-explanatory. You know that prisoners are strong, and they tend to be cunning — so you double-check them at every opportunity. You make sure they don't have trowels to dig their way out, or bars of soap in which to take impressions of pass keys. You try to out-think them at every turn. But what about reversing that, and engaging them in conversation? They are thinking beings aren't they? In which case let's get them agreeing, let's acquire their *consent*.

---

5. Richards, S and Bronson, C (2004), *The Good Prison Guide*, John Blake, pp. 218–245.

It's called dynamic security. It's really only a repeat of the points made about the naughty corner above. If the wrongdoer knows what's involved, acknowledges they've done wrong, and agrees to take the consequences, then you are on a much stronger wicket. They are then using their ineffable human reasoning to work towards the same goal you are—a safer, healthier society. Even in prison, most of those I talked to acknowledged that they had to do their 'time'. Most of them agreed they hadn't really thought things through at the critical time. And I wagered a good many hours of my time that they would jump at the chance to be shown how. As indeed many did. Five years talking things through with people who had the most primitive social skills imaginable—and yet, when time allowed, they flourished. They *consented.* And as Lenny showed beyond doubt, they did arrive at a clear understanding of where they'd gone wrong—and were delighted (and I use that word advisedly) to see it with unexpected clarity.

How you get this through to such as Putin and his ilk is more of a challenge. But if you want *security*, and who doesn't, then the only reliable security you can ever put your faith in is dynamic, that's to say with your client's approval, or, as we have it here, with their *consent.*

In this book, I am trying to convey what worked for me so well in Parkhurst Prison, to the wider society in which we currently find ourselves. Today, we do not have a stable society, either locally or globally. If we are to improve matters, and who could possibly want otherwise, we need clarity, we need to understand where things have gone wrong, and as with all health issues, what is the most therapeutic approach available to us right now. And the model offered here is to label all force, all coercion, all acting without *consent* as essentially infantile, i.e. as a toddler. Transferred unreconstructed from infancy. Force wins when applied to you as a toddler—but, everywhere else, you have to work hard and effectively if you want to survive.

As a doctor, I offer in this book a health-view-of-morality. Underneath layers of *guff*, every single human being ever born wants to be healthier, rather than less. My perception is that for some, as discussed, they have been misinformed to believe that this entails smashing other people into the ground. This operates on an individual scale as with murderers, and on a national or international level, as with demagogues. But in all cases, underneath it all, there is a powerful wish to be healthier.

As before, this needs your *consent* to get anywhere. It wouldn't do to take my word for it. If it is to have any beneficial value at all, then every individual, worldwide, needs to take it on themselves — then there'd be no need for a naughty corner, because there'd be no non-social, unhealthy behaviour to constrain.

CHAPTER 7

Clarity Cures

Murderers' Triple Negatives — Enmity is an Infectious Disease — Every Wrong Person Has Been Wronged — I Spend My Life Taming Electrons, Why Don't You?

Murderers' Triple Negatives

WHAT STRUCK ME MOST ABOUT THE LONG-TERM PRISONERS I worked with was their limited horizons. All right, they had committed the most anti-social act of them all — but, when you got to know them, you found they were only half-human, or more correctly, only half-there. Inside every one of them was a toddler trying to get out, or who had already given up the struggle. As their situation became clearer to me, I summarised it as follows — they had negative social skills, negative self-esteem, and negative futures.

In other words, they asked for what they didn't want, not for what they did. Their social skills were counterproductive — they became very aggressive in their demands, often reinforcing them with violence, or threats of violence. But whatever they got, or indeed had asked for, failed dismally to satisfy. They didn't really want those things. What they wanted was friendliness, respect, to have their *consent* requested. But they had no way of obtaining that. No way of even verbalising it. It was as if they didn't know such social treasures existed. And that, as will be clear from this book, is precisely where the trouble lay — they had never been shown any such social values. They'd never seen them for themselves, in their entire life. Society for them had been uniformly bleak, and the State cemented that in, by imposing on them primitive living conditions, grossly uncivilised routines, amid pronounced anti-social conditions. Negative skill number one — dysfunctional social skills heavily reinforced by the so-called justice system.

Negative self-esteem was even more marked. I well remember one lad, let's call him Tony, who came regularly enough, though he was only half-hearted in his approach. Any notion that he might benefit from seeing me was accompanied by a glaring lack of enthusiasm. Well, since he was there—and since I was up to trying to correct his ennui—on one occasion I decided to be more proactive. I said to him, 'Tony, you think you're rubbish'.

'Yes,' he said. At which point I looked him straight in the eye, and said as forcefully as I could, 'Well I don't. You're not rubbish.' Why not tackle the problem head on, I thought. Well, it didn't work. It had the opposite effect entirely. He leapt to his feet, as if he'd been stung, stormed out of the room, and refused to come and see me again.

Going through the front-door hadn't worked. Even contradicting his self-image, and trying to boost it directly, was counterproductive. It was as if I had mortally offended him. Telling him he mattered alienated him to such a degree that he broke off all contact. I had blown any chance to ameliorate matters, by being too direct, too blunt, too proactive. Not something I would have anticipated, would you?

However, this little story has a happy ending, from an agency I could never have anticipated. At about this time, I was called over to Southampton to be interviewed on the local radio with respect to the work I was doing. In the course of doing so, I related what had happened between me and Tony as an illustration of how difficult it was to break through years of negativity, all of which was being heavily reinforced by the State. We chatted on about other things, and I felt I had managed to convey something of the work I was doing in the prison.

Imagine my astonishment when, later that week, Tony, of all people, coiled himself around the door frame saying sheepishly, 'You were talking about me, weren't you?' Indeed, I was. Courtesy of coincidence, via the local radio, contact was restored, and we set to work with renewed enthusiasm. Our working relationship had been re-cemented. Perhaps it was hearing his story being given public prominence. Perhaps it was acknowledgement that he mattered. I told the public he existed—and this had the beneficial effect that he began to believe it himself. To crown it all, having been illiterate, he then re-commenced his literacy classes—he now had something to live for, something of value out there, following on from uncovering value within himself. His future looked, for the first time in his life, distinctly brighter.

Note carefully how his *negative social skills* cut him off, initially, from any remedy. You can't always rely on a cooperative local radio intervening at the critical time, and this bridging the gap in social skills. Here we were both in luck, which allowed his future to be restored—or even to be introduced for the very first time. Imagine how much *negative non-nutritious emotions* must have been directed at him to produce such an explosive reaction to a single positive comment—can you become allergic to happiness? It would seem so. It is obviously possible to be so damaged socially that you slam the door on any healthier escape route, any remedy, let alone cure—all the more reason for never giving up.

Now to *negative number three*—the future. Why bother to learn to read if your past was dire—and you take this as solid evidence that, along with the present, there's no sensible expectation of change. In fact, on my very first visit to C-Wing, I was struck by how closely these sullen men resembled those in the back wards of the first long-stay hospital I'd worked in 30 years before. Shuffling about, heads down—why look up, when you don't expect to see anything interesting, nor anything you haven't seen a million times before?

Let's bring some clarity into these three negatives. It will come as no surprise that all three fit securely into the kindergarten-view described earlier. No options, no choices, no consents were ever waved in front of them—so there was no way out. Their *nursery nightmares* were here for the duration. Even potentially optimistic input was closed off, as it was with Tony. They had *toddler-vision.* And they had closed the door on anything different, anything better. These three negatives testify to really heavy programming that life for them would always be bad. How many of us are taught this? And how many have an opportunity to lower the drawbridge to let a healthier view in?

Once you see these three negatives, you can detect them all over the place. Take another look at our politicians. Are they exemplars of happily socialising adults? Do they have solid, robust self-esteem? Have they an ongoing and dedicated interest in an ever-brighter future, either for themselves or for the rest of us? If they don't, then what's the likeliest explanation? They've got to the top of the tree, locally at any rate. Why don't they glow in the accolades? Have you noticed how nothing is enough, everything has to be that much bigger, greater, more — nothing slackens the pace. As before, they escalate. And as before, what they ask for doesn't fit. They too have negative social skills — deep enough to account for negative self-esteem and negative futures. Indeed, for them too, the door has been slammed shut. No further intake is possible to fill the emotional black hole they have been left with. Escalation — you see it all over. Invading Poland was not enough. Conquering Russia didn't help. King of the world, but empty inside. Where does this peculiar human grief come from?

And, since we are approaching these issues from a medical viewpoint, where's the remedy? What needs to be brought into the mix to improve matters? What's the cure if there is one? Well, as with all things medical, you need an accurate diagnosis, else all your ministrations will be as water down the drain. Unsurprisingly, the diagnosis offered here is childhoods. Lack of *nutritious emotions* leaves too many with *nursery nightmares*. And, worse, as Tony showed all too clearly, they don't take kindly to having this diagnosis pointed out to them. No, you are just another of those powerful, dreadful people who are meant to offer much, but are never to be trusted.

It goes deep. What I concluded from my explorations of child abuse is that if you are weak and wishy-washy, then not only do you not count for anything, but also your abuser-in-the-head can eat you for breakfast, just as they continue to do themselves. You have to be confident. You have to know what you're doing. You have to be convincing in all these assets. But, as soon as you demonstrate that you're not a pushover, then you move sharply into the dangerous category. If you're strong enough (and adult enough) to defeat any nightmarish figures — then, by that simple fact alone, you are strong enough to repeat the abuse, the trauma, the torture, the reinforcing of a dire view of the world — not an easy conundrum to resolve — but doable, as we now explore.

Enmity is an Infectious Disease

DO NOT TRY AND SHAKE MY HAND, OR HUG ME. Keep well away from me, at least six feet (two metres) or so. I insist you cover your mouth, even though I can't then tell if you're smiling at me or not. And if you're thinking of having a party with people who don't currently live with you, then I shall be forced to send for the police, who will fine you, as they did the then UK Prime

Minster, eventually. It is hard to think of a more devastating way of degrading social health. Yet these laws were enforced to try to limit the number who died, already avoidably high. Covid turned out to be a major killer—and the next pandemic threatens worse.

Yes, you've got to admit, health issues can be really cruel. Even so, the best way to progress is to be as accurate as you can be about what's going on, what you're doing, and why. Exaggeration or lying in this context, for whatever reason, kills. Reality, even if it goes against what you think, has a way of correcting your errors. And if your adversary is a sub-microscopic virus, as with Covid, then you need to be extra considerate, extra vigilant, extra honest—not less. This isn't because I say so, or because I think you are morally corrupt. It's the health-view-of-morality—the more real you are, the healthier you are likely to be. Of course, in this challenging world, there are no guarantees—but if you think about it, which I do, then it stands to reason.

You can't see a virus—in fact no-one knew they existed until electron microscopes came along. Long before that, you could tell an infectious disease by the fact that people who had it gave it to people who hadn't. But you couldn't see the wretched thing which passed from the sick to the healthy. In fact, in the late 1800s, a fierce medical controversy raged as to whether such invisible items could even exist. I still flinch at the fact that male midwives took macho pride in *not* washing their hands between deliveries, with consequences for childbirth-fever you can well imagine, but they could not. So if you think anti-vaxxers are a novelty, then you're in for a surprise—history is full of people who doubt medical evidence, and who do so as if it were a matter of life or death, which it often is.

Sometimes the data is tenuous, as it was when the Covid pandemic first started. This was a new virus. All right, it was related to viruses we had met before, but no-one had immunity against it, because no-one had ever been exposed to it. We were all on a steep learning curve. What we did know was that if you simply didn't breathe the virus in, then you couldn't get the disease. That medical fact stood the test of time. We also knew that immunisation, once it was available, would save us. But the virus tested our social structures, our governing structures, indeed our supplies of *trust* all round—and it did so to the limit. More people died when the *triple values* were deficient. Like I say, *truth, trust* and *consent* matter—not because I say so, or not only because I say so, but because they are the best way that we have of understanding what's happening, what is actually going on in reality—because, like it or not, that's where we all live—and where, when we get it wrong, we die.

The virus for Covid *has always been* invisible—you didn't know if you had it or not. People could infect others without even knowing. Only after symptoms developed could you be clear you had the disease, and could therefore pass it on, passing on a possible death sentence with it. Yes, these are important issues, life is at stake where communal health is involved. It's what stands behind the maxim that no-one-is-safe-until-we're-all-safe, which we fail to learn and implement at our peril.

It became obvious, for clarity's sake, that we needed to know if we were infective or not. How could we tell? The enemy was far too small to be visible with the naked eye, so some other means of detecting it was essential. In short order, along came a number of tests—and most people took to them with glee, working out whether they were a danger to their fellows, by finding if they were positive or not. Another miracle of technology, which sensible Governments made freely available to the populations they were responsible for—and, where they did, fewer died. Yes, health carries the final cut off point—if you are unreal, for whatever reason, then survival rates fall. Testing kits save lives. Efficient, non-corrupt administration keeps more people healthy longer—just as lying, doing things for monetary gain, does the opposite.

We can see micro-organisms with microscopes. Proof that they are there, or not there. If only there was a microscope for the mind, wouldn't that transform mental health? And with it the health of society, and ultimately of peace as opposed to war.

Well attentive readers will already know the answer to that one. Yes, there is a *microscope for the mind*, and there has been for nigh on 30 years. Why, if we take so readily to tests for Covid, has there not been a similar appetite for testing infections of the mind? It's not that one does not exist, so it must be because too many people don't want to look. But since 1995, it has been well-known in medical circles that if you play a trauma tape to someone in a brain scan machine, then parts of their brain cease to show their normal electrical activity. Their electrons are no longer doing what they usually do.

This is not dependent on your philosophy, your point of view, your version of psychiatric theory. No, it's a question of having a look, and thinking about it. If people don't—especially psychiatrists—then something is seriously amiss. What if there were something toxic about trauma, which stopped people thinking straight—what indeed?

We have a pristine, scientific, non-introspective machine telling us if a person's mind isn't fully functional. I'd like to repeat that sentence long enough for its relevance to sink in. For too long it has been fervently believed that the mind is a closed book, it might not even exist. And yet here, for many years, is concrete, objective, scientific evidence not only that some topics close off normal thought, but that 'speechless terror' is real, it happens, it's unhealthy, and people die as a result.

Once the human being stops thinking straight, all sorts of pathologies can accumulate—just from the simple fact that not enough thought is going on to see what damage thoughtlessness is doing. And here we see why enmity is an infective disease. If you don't care that what you do damages people, degrades social health, then you will propagate social disasters without relent. And this is what happens all too often. Drug companies profit from addictive products. Tobacco companies do the same. Media companies make money by peddling enmity. Once you see it, it's obvious—until enough people see it and do something about it, social health suffers.

Fear is the master emotion. And fear underlies hate. When a UK press baron sold more newspapers on the explicit assumption that he intended to give his readers something to hate every day, you would expect two things to follow. Firstly, he would make shedloads of money, and so acquire illegitimate political power. Secondly, he would encourage far too many others to follow his example. Thus, Hollywood and its ilk peddle distrust, under the label of 'jeopardy'. And as for social media today, I think it fair to say that without the malign and neglectful influence of sneer-media, especially Facebook, then the Rohingya who were a substantial Muslim minority in Myanmar (formerly Burma) would not have been expelled from their native country, and found themselves in the biggest refugee camp in the world, in Bangladesh.

Bad news flies around the world, before good news can get her boots on. Fear sells. But it also costs. People pay more attention to a fire that has started, than to one that has been put out. And, as is now a commonplace, eyeballs pay—grab attention, and you make billions. But at what cost? Propagate hate, and social health deteriorates, just as fast or even faster than Covid can spread. Enmity is infectious. And it pays. So somehow more civilised people need to prevail over those addicted to ever more money. Bank balances sound wonderful, but they don't assuage inner emotional chasms. No, for that you need something a great deal less concrete—something which money can never buy—something as shapeless as a *nutritious emotion*. But how would you set about selling one of those? Well, you could start by exploring quite why people go wrong—just where wrong-headedness comes from. Why not start with some simple arithmetic—what could be simpler?

Every Wrong Person Has Been Wronged

IS 2 + 2 = 5, WRONG? 'Of course it is,' you might say, 'every sane person knows that the answer should be 4'. If I raised an eyebrow, you could follow-up by saying—'This is mathematics—the purest, least sullied, most objective form of *science* there is. It's what everybody knows (or should know.) You either accept it, or you're mad.'

But a lot of thinking doesn't actually work like this. Suppose I told you there was a group of people who fervently believed that the answer really was 5, that the world had made a serious mistake, and had been fooled by a whole lot of powerful but misguided people—what then? For the purposes of argument, we could call such people 'Fivists'—they 'knew' 5 was the 'real' answer, and that most people who didn't share that belief were deluded.

We have a divide. On the left, we have people saying the answer is 4, and on the right, that it's 5. How would you decide? Would you take a vote? If the majority said 4, then you could conclude that Fivists were out. Or would you put it to the *scientists*? Ask them to conduct the most scientific experiment they could find, and so decide the matter in a non-subjective, non-introspective and irrefutable manner. If you did that, spare a thought for their difficulties—what you'd probably find is that the best they could manage would be 'market research'—asking as many people as they could get hold of, what they thought the answer should be, and then telling you the result. We call them pollsters, and their findings tend to be more fluid than we'd like.

Then again, some people lie. What if they were covert Fivists, and pretended they weren't. Perhaps they knew they were in a minority, so that they needed to deceive in order to get into high office, such as into the Supreme Court of the USA, widely known by its acronym, SCOTUS.

What happens next? Well, the controversy flares endlessly. There is no answer in the narrow field of simple equations. Some people insist the answer is 5, others that it's 4. Like so many things in life, it would seem to be a matter of opinion. But surely, you might say, mathematics is above belief—you either get it right, or it's you who are in the wrong. However, if you tried this on many controversies you'd get nowhere. Belief is a curious business, and not always a happy one. Putin believed he was right. Alec believed he should spend his energies killing every two years—he didn't think this was wrong. What to do?

Well, the first counter argument is pragmatism. What difference does it make, in practice whether you are a Fivist or not? Suppose every time you added two items to another two you presumed you would get a total of five—what then? The outcome would depend on what you were adding. If it was loaves of bread, and you set about calculating how many (at a loaf a day) you would need for the next five days, then, if your maths was faulty, you'd go hungry, and serve you right. However, if it were something entirely insubstantial, like aesthetics, then little harm would have been done. But note carefully, if you did maintain an 'answer' that a lot of other people told you didn't make sense, then you'd be wise to reconsider. Or at least try out your beliefs in a practical setting—with a fall-back position that was not too drastic.

Which brings us to the second counter argument—health. Does your conviction increase the chances of your being ill, of being unwell, of suffering some sort of disease? Because if it does, then it goes against the health-view-of-morality—the assumption that every human being everywhere wants to live, rather than to die. I've mentioned the group to whom this does not appear to apply—those who think nothing of killing—but the whole thrust of this book is that they are 'wrong', and to prove this, given enough resources of a special, and for them an unusual, kind they will, like Alec did, come round to our common more *realistic* view.

Let's take a really contentious issue such as abortion. How would you balance this out? Well, on a health-view-of-morality, you would consider the question factually. Leaving aside hot emotions, and a bunch of distorting statements, while trying to provide a thoroughly rinsed statement—one you would expect from an involved but dispassionate doctor, try this: 'The world would be a healthier place if you allowed every fertilised human egg to grow to full maturity and come into a world in which its parents didn't want it.' Agree or disagree?

But hang on a minute—this was meant to be a leisurely discussion of how 'wrongness' worked, first in mathematics, a dry and unemotional topic, and then by extension, crime, violence and war. And yet here we are in one of the hottest, most controversial topics of the day, recently ignited by a self-opiniated SCOTUS, and inflaming the whole world. How did this come about? Well, all I can say is that the process of writing is infinitely mysterious—you have an idea in mind, words tumble out, you sort through them as through a pack of cards, discarding those which don't fit in smoothly, while retaining that which adds something, especially something of zest. Since the issue of SCOTUS came up, out popped the loaded issue of abortion—and being comfortably placed at this point, I did not immediately censor it, but allowed it to stand, and decided I would need to explore how to weave it into the text, without alienating a chunk of my readers.

Now I have not the least intention of deciding this point for you. There are a lot of challenging questions in this world, not all of which have simple, or enduring answers. It is not for me to decide for you. But it is my task to encourage you to think. To look at the problem from as many angles as are available to you, and then to weigh things up as equitably as you can. Suppose you came to my clinic asking whether you should have an abortion or not. What would I do? Well, the first thing would be to put you at your ease—these are hot issues, and much gets melted in the heat. Once you were sitting comfortably, I would carefully explore with you what your personal views were. Had you considered all the implications? I would not be seeking to persuade you either way—no, my job would be to sort through the various options available, none of which might seem ideal.

Having ascertained what your current thinking was, I would bring into the discussion points which you might have missed. Had you thought through adoption? Did you, fully, take into account the fact that you were now in a position to give birth to a new person, who would have to face our difficult world for many decades? Are you aware of how critical the first few years of life are to later happiness, or health? Is there social, marital or domestic support available to you? And if there is, is it, in your view, sufficient? And if it's not, does this alter what's in your mind?

What this digression into abortion is meant to show is that thinking things through in as calm and rational way as possible is how we clever human beings solve the innumerable problems which life, especially social life, throws at us. When we came into this world, we were not guaranteed a quiet or calm passage through it — many things can trip us up, and we, all of us, need help, support, even *nutritious emotions*, to get through.

The fact of the matter is that starting a whole new life, as with a new-born, just highlights the entirely inexplicable wonder of what life is really about. We don't know where it comes from. We can pull a few strings to improve it — but fundamental to that is concerted social action, something that is not always easy to achieve. Emotions can cripple, but clarity can cure. At least that's my sterling conviction. And what is even more remarkable is when you get clarity on the very substance of which we are composed, the wonder and delight increase. Or they do for me as I will now try and expound.

I Spend My Life Taming Electrons — Why Don't You?

ELECTRONS DO EXACTLY WHAT I TELL THEM TO. If I order them to come, they come. If I insist that they go, they go. *I am living proof that the* uncertainty principle *does not apply to me.* I add this emphasis because I want it to outrage any dyed-in-the-wool *scientist* who might read it. If you are a fervent believer in the Great Science Illusion mentioned in *Chapter 4*, then I would not be a bit surprised if you now drop the book in horror, and conclude that this time I really have gone too far — I must be talking nonsense.

For those who are brave enough to continue thinking, I can say, with absolute *certainty*, that within the next micro-second, you too will tame electrons in exactly the same way I do. Within a matter of minutes, you will have pressed an electric switch. And, if you're still prepared to go against the heavy weight of conventional wisdom, you will know that this act of yours tells the electrons to stop doing what they were doing and start doing the opposite. You control them to such a degree that they do what you want, not what they want.

Suppose the switch in question is a light switch. Do you want extra photons in the room? Then press it. Do you want less? Then press it again. What is causing the change? Who is deciding to flood the place with utterly unknowable photoelectrons? What brought about the dramatic change? Well, you did. You were the one who did the switching, no-one else. The electrons certainly didn't. They took absolutely no part in the decision.

And look at the *certainty* with which you did it. So much so that you didn't even think twice. The room in your judgement is getting a little dark, so you have reached out and pressed the light switch before it even occurs to you that that's what you needed to do. What I'm asking you to do is pause, think, and just look at what that means to the general scheme of things. It means you have absolute control over how many photoelectrons you permit in the immediate space around you. You say, they do. If they don't, if the switch doesn't work, if no extra electrons obey your command, you don't collapse in a heap and say the inherent chaos of the inanimate cosmos has defeated you all over again. You don't despair that the *uncertainty of things* has won again—no, you change the fuse, you pay the electric bill, you correct the engineering fault, and get on with the rest of your life, as if it were the most natural thing in the world, which of course it is.

What makes the difference? You don't need a Large Hadron Collider, like the one in Switzerland smashing zillions of subatomic particles—but you do need to be awake, or at least alive. Because somehow, in a manner I have no intention of exploring further, being alive redirects electrons. Nothing moves without them, so when you move, you use them, not them you. And you use them to breathe with. Which is where that astonishing oxygen comes in—it swaps electrons about. I don't know how it does this, I doubt very much that anyone really does—but I do know that carbohydrates are fuel which when combined with oxygen give out energy, as in any combustion device, and—wait for it—as in any living organism.

Yes, that's right. Living organisms burn fuel. They trap electrons and put them to work. Electrons then operate your chest muscles to enable to you breathe. When they stop, so do you. Here particle physics underwrites health. You cannot be healthy if the electrons in you cease to do what you want, and start misbehaving in a thoroughly chaotic way, like they do in the wild. And that last word gives the game away. Electrons in lightning or anywhere else are wild. They do act without pattern, at random, without meaning, without organization. It's only living organisms that have found a way of organizing them. Don't ask me why. Nor have I any interest in how they do this—but

I am desperate to ensure that they do it, and that they continue doing so for as long as is feasible. Because non-thinking humans seem intent on drawing the whole miraculous process to a halt—thermonuclear radiation restores the primeval chaos, from which we, and all other living entities, have laboriously and painstakingly emerged.

Now, let's put a little mystery back into the *uncertainty principle*. *Uncertain* is right, and will always remain so. And to show just how miraculous organisms are, let's look at the simplest proof that uncertainty is here to stay. Quantum physics usually closes the mind because it's impossible to understand—well here's one feature of it, and a fundamental one at that, which you, they, or even a young child will find simple, obvious, and entirely understandable. Again, not the usual attributes of subatomic physics.

The foundations of physics, and therefore of *science* in general, began to go pear shaped in 1900. A remarkable scientist found to his surprise that electricity, and energy in general, was not what we thought. We talk gaily of electric circuits. We say electric current flows. But this is only part of the truth. If you get down to the nitty-gritty, energy is not continuous, it comes in packets, called quanta. Small parcels of 'energy', not streams of it. They come in such profusion that they behave like a stream, but when you look closely enough, they're not.

Now we all know about parcels. And if energy is fundamentally parcel shaped, then we're in trouble. If it behaved like a wave, then we can tell when it is likely to arrive—if it's a metre away, and travelling towards us at a metre a second, then it'll be here in one second's time. But if it's a parcel, we can never be certain. A parcel, as with postal deliveries, sets out, takes its time travelling, and may arrive sooner, or later, 'depending'—each parcel being independent of the channel along which it is conveyed. We never doubt this with the real-life parcel post—and there's no way round it with subatomic parcels or quanta either. It doesn't help that these little rascals sometimes behave like a wave, when we call them a 'wave-particle'. Nor is it helpful for our understanding when they seem to be in two places at once, nor even influence each other at a distance—all very *uncertain*—which goes to show just how unexpected, delightful and astonishing living organisms, such as ourselves, are. We, and they, can, and continuously do, control the final product—goodbye *uncertainty*—at least so long as we're alive.

Well, this is such a profoundly different take on life, on decisions, intentions, choices that it has impact not only on philosophy, and on health as indicated, but also on economics, politics and, the pinnacle we are aiming for here, sanity. If living organisms organize electrons, some do so better than others. Humans are a social species, so they do better by being sociable, by cooperating. Combining energies means we can do more. And devising symbols or tokens of 'organizing' can facilitate joint efforts beyond recognition. We call it money, but what coinage really measures is how much we have deployed our ability to control electrons to increase order, and thereby reduce disorder. The technical term for disorder is 'entropy'. In everyday language we'd call it 'chaos'.

Now chaos is unhealthy. On this definition, it's electrons doing what they do, and not what we want them to do. It is also related to economic activity. This opens a topic too large for this page—but one which is desperately needed when social health is at stake. Billionaires cannot really have earned that amount, if you relate economic value to organizing-ability. Electron-control links to money in a fascinating way, but it's one that will have to wait for another day.

What does apply here is sanity. If I can control electrons, then am I going to do so in a manner which helps you? Or not. And what makes the difference? The point being, can we put flesh on the maxim—no-one-is-sane-until-we're-all-sane? Here's where the closing chapter hopes to go.

CHAPTER 8

A-Smile-a-Day-Keeps-the-Doctor-Away

What's in a SMILE?—Oh No, It is an Ever Fixéd Mark—Sanity is Our Only Social Reality—Is JOY Only Ever for Other People?

What's in a SMILE?

WHAT EXACTLY IS A 'SMILE'? First define (or at least try to describe) your terms. In this final chapter, I need to reverse the writer's normal approach. Up to this point in the book, I have been at pains to encourage the reader to the view that they know more than at first appears, that everyday life does indeed offer more solutions than is generally supposed, and that, yes, there is a simplicity underlying the obvious chaos.

Here, however, I find I need to do the opposite. With a smile, I am in the position of having to point out the reader's ignorance—not trivial ignorance, but deep, permanent, and ineradicable ignorance. In other words, there are aspects of the smile which you think you understand, that you fondly believe you know well enough—yet it's now my challenging duty to disabuse you of such a comfortable notion, and to point out to you, as convincingly as I possibly can, that you are mistaken. Generally speaking, that's a sure fire way of losing the interest of readers altogether—pointing out that they actually know far less than they think they do—a recipe for diminishing readers' enthusiasm, for reducing their self-confidence, and for diluting what because of my writing may be an already tenuous attention span.

Nevertheless, that's precisely what a smile demands that I now do. More, I must also couple this ignorance-emphasis with a request that, at this point, you do something extra, something that will interrupt your current comfortable reading posture, and *move*. For the opening of this final chapter, you are required to put the book down for a moment and reach for the nearest mirror.

121

Like all sensible writers, I am fully aware that the channel of communication between me and you can easily become clogged. The words I have available to me are clumsy, they crumble all too easily when called upon to do more than they can. They offer decidedly more than they can guarantee to deliver. I entertain a delicious notion that what I write makes sense, that it conveys a meaning which does expand the reader's view, gives them a new 'take' on something they previously thought was entirely familiar. Well, stand by whilst I undertake a more challenging verbal task than usual — the opposite. Try the following.

Now once you've located the nearest mirror, smile at it. What could be simpler? The corners of your mouth go up, there are little wrinkles that appear around your eyes, and your whole face lights up. Or does it? This is what the mirror is for. Look closely again. And then repeat. At first you might find yourself smiling in a natural fashion. But press it, as I must now request you do, and the smile promptly degrades into a grin. Of course, you can pretend. You can make-it-up. You can smile when you don't really mean it — and there you have the point of these opening paragraphs. There is something in the smile which is *spontaneous*. It is unique. It is ephemeral. But it is also vital. It shows an aspect of being alive which mere words struggle to attain. A 'real' smile is something wonderful, it is invariably delightful, it warms your heart, it makes you want to live.

Now just look at those four positive attributes, digest them, and you have in your grasp as full an understanding of what this book is about as I can give you. Your smile matters to you. It contains within, qualities I can only refer to obliquely via these static words. It's alive, whereas, once I've written them, they're not. By looking at how your mouth moves, how your facial muscles 'join in' — all this contributes to the indescribable mystery of a smile. I cannot capture in printed words what you can so easily observe in real life. I can refer to it. I can prescribe a variety of things that I can invite you to do — but your smile is your own, you are in charge of it, and you can deliver it, or withhold it, at your entire discretion.

Except that there is a crucial, and elusive aspect of the smile, which defies all these things. You *cannot* fully control it. If you do, your smile is contrived, and its impact sullied. 'Smile, smile, and yet be villain' — as the poet has it. A false smile is worse than none at all. So here we have the *triple values* creeping in again. *Truth, trust* and *consent* are intrinsic to warm, genuine smiles — and where they're absent, the smile goes cold — a most unpleasant experience.

But back to the warmth of a natural smile. It comes on by itself. It opens up your face and your mind to a benignity which can only do good. You look across the room at your companion and you give her or him a smile. What has happened? 'What gives?' as they say. Well, something cheerful has occurred. Something that wasn't there before lifts the atmosphere. It says, 'It's all right, I'm on your side, I won't attack you, I enjoy being in your company.' Well, you can see I'm struggling here a little, hoping to capture in cold print something that is intrinsically fluid. And that's the crux — being fluid is one thing, but flowing in a benign direction is extra. And this is precisely what we all desperately need — our thoughts can flow all over the place — but this very fluidity needs directing. We can so easily get lost in our own chunterings — a smile can say, 'This direction is preferred over that.' A smile gives a pointer, a helpful pointer. It says this is safer, this is better, this is good. And how many things do that for you, or for me?

Like so many pre-clinical medical students, and others, I was desperately keen to understand how the human mind works. I read as widely as I could. And I took a course in psychology, in one of the world's leading universities. And I was short-changed. The pioneering professor followed the fashion of the day — and studied rats. He couldn't afford chimpanzees, he didn't have the emotional confidence to look more closely at humans, so he counted how fast rats ran, in artificially constructed mazes. What a calumny. I mention this, because the most striking phrase which comes to me from that year was one I heard in the film, *Some Like It Hot*. In it, our hero exhorts his friend to smile at a possible benefactor. In order to advance their status in life, he says, 'Don't just smile — give him the teeth, the whole personality.' Which he does, to fruitful effect all round.

But look at that expansion of the smile. Showing the teeth in a smile increases its weight, its impact, its meaning. How can a smile have weight? More — how can it have impact? And where does 'meaning' come into it? Well, it does. I can write this down. I can ask you to agree. But, as with the mirror just now, only if you see for yourself, see the whole process in action, can you begin to feel the full effect of a smile.

And it's worth the effort. A smile tells you things about the person you are in contact with, that mere words do not. Poets capture more, or can capture more, than ordinary prose writers. But nothing can compare with lived experience. It's a bit like breathing. You breathe in and out as if there was nothing to it. You smile, or receive a smile, as if this was entirely normal. But in both cases, there is far more going on than immediately hits the eye. And to emphasise quite how much — all that has to happen is for either to stop. Discomfort from choking is immediate and agonising, whereas absence of smiles, though harder to pin down, chokes off the mind almost as much.

Lack of oxygen has a parallel in active sneers, or frowns. If you think I am exaggerating just how vital smiles are to the health of the mind, then consider sneers, frowns, grimaces, and scowls. These are active negative emotions. Again, you may have difficulty defining precisely what they are. You may also have equivalent problems in repeating them into your mirror — you can pretend them, just as you could the smile earlier — but the real thing hits deeper. And if it comes from someone who matters to you, then the impact can be devastating. And lasting.

It is no exaggeration to say that smiling helps you keep sane, whereas scowling does the opposite. We are creeping up on unpacking the maxim no-one-is-sane-until-we're-all-sane, and this is another way of gaining the same point. You can smile at yourself in the mirror. Or you can receive a *spontaneous* smile from someone who is significant to you — and when you do, your mind lights up in exactly the same way their face does — which moves the discussion a bit further towards a-smile-a-day-keeps-the-doctor-away.

Oh No, It is an Ever Fixéd Mark

I MAKE NO APOLOGY at this point, for reaching deeper into poetry. The fluidity of the mind can be its greatest asset — we can conjure up trips to the moon, as easily as imagining our next delicious meal. But we also crave stability. We need something to anchor our fleeting thoughts to, else our mental world decomposes into a discomforting whirl. When you read in a well-known poem that the poet has found an 'ever fixéd mark', it pays to pay attention — What is this? Where does it come from? And can I have some, please?

So, let's take those three questions in order. First, what is it? Well, if you accept the poet's word for it, it is 'love'. But, sadly for the present era, this four-letter word has acquired as many meanings as a box of snakes—which is why I didn't brandish it in the prison. All words wander about, their meanings varying from time-to-time, and from place-to-place. Even within the same speaker the words can vary following one experience or another. The one thing that is consistent throughout is being alive, which is why I place so much on the health-view-of-morality. I cannot overemphasise the fact that though humans are immeasurably different the world over—and indeed next door—the one thing they can unite around is health. Of course, there are many versions of what even this medically-based word means, but there's one point they all have in common—delaying, deferring, putting off the inevitable, otherwise known as death.

Poets are allowed special licence, special flexibility with words—they can bend them, squeeze them, re-invent them, spread them wider than normal prose or conversation allows. In Shakespeare's case, he being the poet in question, we can expect extreme liberties—indeed we relish them. It's like watching an accomplished acrobat throw himself or herself through the hoops with gay abandon, always landing safely on the other side. Indeed, we thrill at the way he or she sets problems for themselves, and then solves them with a fluidity that makes us gasp. There are times when their meaning is not as clear as it might be—but there are so many others when the acrobat points us to a part of humanity that we hadn't really looked at as closely as we might before.

This is what Shakespeare does with 'love'. Not only does he tackle the inherent shapelessness of this word, but he does so, on this occasion, within the rigid framework of a sonnet. Now a sonnet must consist of 14 lines, each of ten syllables, only 140 in all. The lines must rhyme alternately, except the last couplet, which rhymes with itself. What it does on this occasion, is intrigue us—we ponder why he expresses himself quite in this way, why not in another? He makes what appear to be outrageous statements, and then embroiders them. We can gain a glimpse of his thinking, what mattered to him, and how he approached the many imponderables of life—and we do so, even after a gap of over 400 years—quite remarkable.

This line is from Sonnet 116. I remember reading this as an adolescent, struggling with falling in love, or not—and being nicely sceptical of his earlier protestation that 'Love is not love which alters when it alteration finds.' In my then experience, love was regularly altering whenever it felt like it—indeed, it seemed to do so on purpose. Stability, reliability, consistency were at a premium (and still are)—so the poet here was talking through his hat. I even remember saying as much to my then girlfriend, though I don't recall this helping.

And then we have to detach 'love' from sex. In Jane Austen's day—'She made love to me in the hall' would evoke a different frisson than nowadays. She meant something rather less earthy than we gasp at today. And, medically speaking, sex seems to cause as many problems as it solves. People fret they are not having enough, that it doesn't last long enough, and that when sexual attraction wanes then that's the end. None of which seems to trouble Shakespeare in the least. In fact, much angst has been spilt over whether he was addressing his poetry to a woman or a man. We'd perhaps make more progress, and gain more from him, if we allow him to be gender neutral—something that every infant certainly is.

If we rinse love of its many misunderstandings, we can focus on it being the relationship between two human beings of indeterminate gender. Shakespeare insists that though one might get older, and presumably more wrinkled, love itself, in this context, does not alter. He clearly sees how two humans can grow a bond between themselves, which survives 'tempests', the passage of time, and even 'the edge of doom'. Whatever it is, it sounds wonderful—we'd all like some, so to the second question—where does it come from?

Shakespeare starts off by imposing an overblown idealistic condition onto the rest of his sonnet. He demands a 'marriage of true minds'. And of course, if you can acquire a couple of those, then you're in clover. So that's where it comes from—true minds married together.

Indeed, that could be the motto for all of us—let's find enough 'true minds' to provide us with the stability and security that we all yearn for, and indeed need. Sanity is not possible without them. Shakespeare asserts that such a thing is possible. I agree. Not everyone does. The question arises, why not? And the answer in this book is because we've never learnt, we've never been taught that minds can be true for long enough to allow all parties to 'look on tempests and never be shaken'. My words are not as obedient as his—ah well, I'll just do-what-I-can-with-what-I've-got.

What Shakespeare doesn't do is look for the answer by ever closer study of nature, nowadays called *science*. Indeed, in a different sonnet, Number 18, he has the redolent phrase 'Nature's changing course untrimmed'. This acknowledges that 'nature', or the world around us, keeps changing all by itself—later called chaos, or entropy—yet, according to Shakespeare, humans can 'trim' it. That is to say, they can nudge it one way rather than another. And if they can once do that, then there's no limit to the problems they can resolve. War, peace, sanity—all fall within our compass—so why don't we do it?

So to the third question—can I have some, please? Now this does raise serious questions. First, we'd have to agree that such a thing as an 'ever-fixéd-mark' does or can exist. And there are many, even quite eminent philosophers, who are happy to convince you that it doesn't and can't. Here's where belief stops you seeking anything further. And why an unusual phrase, such as no-one-is-sane-until-we're-all-sane, does not immediately roll off the tongue as the most natural thing in the world. But here we are being driven by the impending threat of Nucleargeddon, so there is extra pressure on us to push the envelope, extend the boundaries of orthodoxy in the hope of gaining something more durable, and less liable to fossilise us all.

And if a smile is difficult to capture in words, then peace-of-mind is perhaps harder still. But 'true minds' gives a clue, just as a smile points towards benignity. And if you are relating to another, to a mind which seems to be married to yours, at least in certain respects, and now and again, then you are on the right lines to achieve a reliable, repeatable, and ever healthier state of mind.

I like the adjective 'true'. It relates, in my book, to the degree to which your account, your picture of what's happening around you, actually matches the reality. Because it does take a measure of confidence to acknowledge that we will never know with absolute certainty just what that reality consists of—and even if we did, we'd be out of date all too quickly.

I suppose it could be called a measure of philosophical humility. I, you, or we can never know 100% what's going on. We have to do the best we can—and call on as many resources as are available to us at that time—in other words, on other minds, especially those that are 'true', and to which we can be 'married', if only from time-to-time.

And if you're interested in mental stability, in mental security, in self-confidence, then all these emotive phrases converge on the notion of sanity, to which we now turn.

Sanity is Our Only Social Reality

INSANITY IS A DEFICIENCY DISEASE. And until this redolent fact sinks in, doctors will continue to make a hash of it, just as they did with scurvy before some bright spark suggested you suck lemons. If you're ill, the first thing you think of is—'What's causing it, where did it come from, was it something I ate?' External factors are the easiest to understand. You broke your leg because you fell. You got Covid, because you breathed an infected person's air. You couldn't get it without. Had you not been exposed to the injurious agent, you'd have remained well.

As a medical student you have it drummed into you that disease has a whole range of causes—you rattle them off in order to pass your exams—seven varieties, if I remember correctly. These range from what you're born with it, what you're infected by, even, for the more sophisticated, what drugs you're taking. Always stuff that was done to you, not something that wasn't.

And for the most part it works well enough. Of course, it makes eminent sense. Disease after disease fell to this 'external' model. One of the most dramatic was malaria. What possible connection could this often-fatal disease have to a small, biting insect? Well, none of course, at least none that meets the eye, the naked eye at that—until one intrepid doctor, toiling away with one of these new-fangled microscopes, in the outback, was looking at, of all things, a mosquito's entrails. There he actually saw, in the gut of these tiny bloodsucking insects, wriggling organisms which matched exactly those in an infected person's blood. Sounds like witchcraft—blood of toad, eye of newt, and all that—but it has saved innumerable lives. Sleep behind a net, and unlike those around you, you will not get malaria. Powerful stuff.

Nor is it easy to introduce something which goes against the conventional wisdom. So many 'old-wives-tales' need debunking that yet another one is easily dismissed. If you are outlandish enough to prescribe something as amorphous as a 'smile', then you must expect the devastating weight of medical scepticism to dog your days—as it did.

Yet other deficiency diseases, even deadlier than scurvy, do occur. Whisper it carefully, but the leading cause of death worldwide—heart disease—could be coming from something we're not doing. No, just bear with me, and go back to basics—see if simplification here can shed any light, as it has done before. What do you lose when your heart stops working? What should your heart be doing, before it became ill? Well, it pumps blood around your body, everyone knows that. Your heart works harder if you do more. Exercise stretches your circulatory system so that it can cope with more than if you sit around all day long. So perhaps that old adage applies here too—use it or lose it.

Look at the history. In the 1890s heart attacks were a medical rarity. Doctors would hurry to the bedside of a patient with a coronary—you didn't see one every day, so you needed to make the effort. Not so nowadays. What's changed? Well before the motor car, everyone walked, or rode bouncing horses—very energetic. You didn't expect to sit back in your limo. No, if you wanted to go somewhere else you had to work at it, and work hard. Those horses took some riding on, if you didn't want to fall off. And Shank's Pony stretched your walking legs, as a matter of course.

Let's be equally concrete about the mind. What is it for? What should it be doing before it becomes ill? And could it also be that the less you use it the more you lose? And here we hit our first problem. No-one nowadays doubts that the heart is a pump, and that the blood *circulates*. Shakespeare didn't know this. Harvey hadn't told the world—so no-one then knew. But now you don't get medically ostracised for saying so.

The mind, however, is a different kettle of fish. First of all it's possible to pretend it doesn't really exist—not a good start if you want to know where it goes wrong. Next, even if you assert that we all have a mind, and we start using it before, or immediately after, we're born, like Ethan did in *Chapter 2*—there's no universal agreement about what you use it for. And assertions that it's the organ of socialising tend to fall on deaf ears. And when you go further, and insist that it's central asset is the ability to dream up things that were never there before—well what can you expect?

It's like trying to define 'spontaneity'. Definitions rely on relating that item to something that's happened before—and yet being spontaneous is precisely doing something which has only just come into existence. Which makes consciousness the most intriguing entity in our entire cosmos, bar none. We use it every day, even every minute. We think things through. The room is getting darker, we work out why, and then take remedial action. We can even solve problems we've never had to face before, such as viral pandemics spread by air travel. And we conjure up ways of going about it, that were entirely novel. They had to be. If they'd been just the same as before, we'd be dead.

Spontaneity is the key. Which rather puts paid to the efforts of both Pavlov, and indeed Freud. Their endeavour was to find rules which would govern what happened next. Pavlov's dogs would salivate when he rang the bell — all he needed to do was to find the right 'bell' and all human behaviour would fall into place. He was looking to turn us into machines — you'd only need to ring the appropriate bell and we'd salivate. Freud too, sought the *science of the mind* — he started by having 'sex' as the fuel which drove it, and he wasn't deterred by the fact that he kept needing to move on from the genitals, to the anus, the breast, and even a nonsense like a 'life-death' instinct. No, sorry, *science* cannot predict what hasn't been thought up yet. And thank goodness it can't — it's being *spontaneous* that makes life worth living, or indeed keeps us from dying.

Having had a punt at what the mind is, what's it for? Well, thinking up solutions to the incessant problems which our inanimate, and chaotic world insists on throwing at us keeps it up to scratch. It 'solves' things. That's what it's for. Fancy having to put that in writing. Except, it's what everyone does, every minute of every day. The room becomes too dark, we switch on the light. We don't even think about it — but note carefully, if we were unable to think, then no light would ever be switched on.

We can see for ourselves the darkness or lightness of a room. But there are even more vital things for which we need help. These are things we cannot discern for ourselves. And there's an awful lot of them. Not only that, but they are the most important things of all. Again, I don't fancy defining them, and these pesky words, which are all I've got at my disposal, really make even trying to describe them an uphill task. Smiles you can see readily enough — but trying to capture them in cold print is something else. When it comes to peace-of-mind, you're really pushing it.

But again, we are a social species. Smiles cement friendship. They also point the way towards a better way of going about things. If you have confirmation that what you're about to do is sensible, and likely to make things better rather than worse, then that's precisely what you need. Smiles can do this. Social confirmation goes deeper than you might think. Indeed, on this thread, sanity is being confirmed by everyone else. Hence — no-one-is-sane-until-we're-all-sane. Insanity, in this view, is being out of sync with reality. Things are going on out there that you have not taken into account. Your view of the world outside is out-of-date. You can no longer rely on what you think you know to get you through. Our chaotic world is changing all the time — the weather is the least of it. We need up-to-date info to guide us to a resolution. Unless we resolve things, we're done for.

Every living organism needs to keep tabs on what's really happening out there. If it doesn't, it dies. Not because I say so, not because it's a wicked world — it's the Law of Life — adapt, keep in touch, keep real, or perish. Which is the sole purpose of having a mind in the first place. Only by puzzling how it does it, can we begin to see where it goes wrong. And only then can we uncover sure fire ways of putting it right.

Is JOY Only Ever for Other People?

SHARE A LOAF, AND IT'S HALVED — *BUT* SHARE AN IDEA, AND YOU'VE *DOUBLED* IT. It's the same with smiles — the more you give, the more you get. That splendid Yorkshire saying comes close — 'Money is like muck (farmyard manure)…it's no good, unless it's spread around'. But just a minute, this is serious. How can this be? Give something away, and you get more? It doesn't make a lot of sense. We all know that if you have two potatoes, and you donate one, that halves your food stock — there will only be 50% left out of what there was before. It's elementary kindergarten logic — it's what we've all learned all too deeply since we were small. What's yours is yours, what's mine is mine — and what I eat, you can't. Having your cake *and* eating it is the classic no-no from nursery times.

Are we going to leave it there? There's only so much to go around, and once it's gone, it's gone? Well, not if you look that bit deeper. And — watch this one closely—not if you go out into the garden, or onto the farm. Here you find things growing. Yes, you plant a small seed, and a whole new plant springs into existence. Here your investment miraculously expands. Which is quite fortunate, since without food crops we and our livestock would starve. You might have difficulty digesting the notion that without sharing thoughts, beliefs and ideas our mental world is impoverished—but no-one can deny that without planting seeds, or harvesting crops, we wouldn't last the winter. Things grow in the soil—we don't really know how, but we couldn't survive if they didn't. All I'm suggesting is that things grow in the mind, along the same lines.

So, let's take a closer look at plants. What do they do all day? Well, they sit around absorbing solar energy, turning it into carbohydrates and other wonders, which we then munch through to our hearts' (and stomachs') content. Yes indeed. Photosynthesis—don't you just love it? So come with me, while we explore, briefly, the Quantum Life of Plants—that's to say, how our everyday plants cope with quanta.

In the 1920s, the *uncertainty principle* told us that you could never know both where an electron is, *and* where it's going—you had to choose—either where it now is, or how fast it's moving away, never both at the same time. Uncertainty was built into the subatomic world. But no-one told the plants. They cheerfully gobble up all those *uncertain* solar photoelectrons, as if it were the most natural thing in the world. They don't seem to understand that you can never ever tell when a quantum will arrive, or how it can be in two places at once, or whether light is really a wave or a particle. They don't care. They just keep harvesting solar power, binding carbon dioxide with water, giving us glorious nutritious food. Do I really need to point out that animals don't photosynthesise? Solar energy rots our skin. We can't eat sunbeams. If all our plants died off, as they did 65 million years ago when dust clouds from that meteor strike shut off the sunshine, then we'd be starved into extinction, just like the dinosaurs. The crocodiles didn't mind—they thrive on cadavers. Will they feast on ours?

Therefore, if plants can tame electrons, why can't we? Let's stop thinking of electrons as random, chaotic hostiles, and look on them as allies. Radical? I should say so. But elementary. Watch closely as I explore how we couldn't survive without them.

In the last chapter, I stressed that *I'm living proof that the* uncertainty principle *doesn't apply to me.* I anticipated that dyed-in-the wool scientists would drop the book in horror and throw mud and other calumny at me from the sidelines — it's the way they've been trained. But in real life, electrons do what I tell them to — I couldn't lift a cup to my lips without them. And since I do, as a matter of course, it never occurs to me that I can't — I tame electrons as if that were the most natural thing in the world. And so do you — though perhaps with less conviction, at least to begin with. The health-view-of-morality requires nothing less.

If you wish to keep living, then I recommend breathing in and out — and the only way you can do this is to activate your respiratory muscles, which wouldn't move an inch unless you could supply adequate numbers of tamed electrons to power them forwards. Again, most people do this without a second thought — which is a shame, because if you think about it, it's quite miraculous that such unruly particles, or wave-particles, or whatever, stand between you and not-you. You couldn't exist without them, so don't try.

You could even develop a soft spot for such life-saving electrons — though I wouldn't recommend getting too emotionally involved, because there's another batch coming along in your next meal. And should you, for any reason, doubt the vital role they play, then I suggest you call into service a splendid gizmo called an electro-myo-gram (EMG). Put one in position, hold your breath as long as you can, then breathe — and this little gadget will record electrons rushing around like billyo, doing precisely what you'd expect them to do.

Moving on, once these vital electrons have been tamed, what should you do with them? Well keeping you alive is a good starter — but then what? Some use them to invade Ukraine — but to do that, you have to have a remarkably robust method of not-thinking-things-through. But before things become too complex, it's best to get down to basics.

Simplifying things to begin with makes it easier to grasp subtleties later. So here we need to call on Ethan again (*Chapter 2*). There he was, unable to smile, since it would take him a couple of months to gain control of his facial musculature. But his tongue was his to do with as he wished. Had it not been, he could never have ingested enough calories to 'burn' with the oxygen he so recently started breathing in, so as to power the electrons which moved his tongue where he wanted.

He conversed with his dad. All right, sticking your tongue out is rather a primitive way of communicating with your fellows — but if it's all you've got, then best make as full use of it as you can. Which he does. More, he 'converses' with every audience I get to show the video to. And, as you can imagine, I show it at every opportunity I can muster. And one of the main reasons I do so is to hear the collective, 'Aaaaawh' that goes up whenever he performs. What is actually happening? What are these people responding to — he's only been born a few minutes, and off they go — the ones that are awake that is?

They are socialising with Ethan. And socialising delights them — enough smiles and you get delight, enough delights and you get joy — if you can. Which brings us to my delight with Alec. Here's the other thing I also show whenever I can — it's Alec demonstrating in a remarkable way that clarity cures. The *clarity* in this case coming via his mother. Just read this through, so you can see why it delights me:

'A 254 Bob: Mmm, I say to people, and I hope this doesn't upset you, I say to people that you would have been a serial killer.

A 255 Alec: Yeah, yeah, and I believe that's true, there's no doubt about that.

A 256 Bob: There isn't is there?

A 257 Alec: I know what would have happened. But like I said I was lucky, all right I didn't feel that way at the time, but now I know that I was lucky, I was lucky to be put in here [C-Wing, Special Unit, Parkhurst Prison]. If I had been put in a different unit, which at the time that's what I wanted, the same thing would have still happened. Not this — the violence, you know. And really I've the governors, especially the governors of Moorland and G, to thank for bringing me here.

And you know, my mum on the visit, she said you've really matured, you've really like, suddenly from being like a kid and being all like teenagery and all that, you've just wiped that out, she says and now you can see the seriousness in your face when you're talking about things. She says you put yourself across, whereas I know before you couldn't do that. And she admitted, she said, I suppose, I'll be honest, she says I'm to blame. But she says, now, I know different, and I know now how to talk to you, she says, and give you the respect, as an adult, that you deserve. She says I know that I've overpowered you, and yeah and I have clung on to you. She says, but

now while we're not seeing each other, I can get hold of my life now and
know that you are ...
A 258 Bob: She said that?
A 259 Alec: Yeah.
A 260 Bob: *She* can get on with *her* life? Ha ha ha!'

As you might expect, I see this as Alec ridding himself of all his *toddler-
thinking*. For me, his mother's endorsement of his mature, adult face confirms
it. Reading this now, 30 years later, even brings a tear to my eye — what a thing
are emotions! And when other people delight in it, it does actually bring me joy.

So, joy comes courtesy of other people. It takes a degree of emotional confidence to see it. And it is actually a by-product of taming those electrons. We
delight when we tame them. We also delight in others, when they do sports,
gymnastics, ballet, art, music, dance, theatre — each and every human activity
which shows to each of us how others, too, can tame electrons — that's a wow,
that's a delight, and if you get enough of it, that's a joy.

People will find their own source. For me, one of my more reliable sources
of immeasurable delight is Schubert. I don't play him well, but his piano duets
carry me to a pinnacle, to an acme of human creativity and delight. My organ-
ist friend says that playing Schubert's piano duets is a privilege, which it is. But
then so is being alive — wouldn't you agree?

APPENDICES

1. Supporting References
2. George Orwell's Review of *Mein Kampf* (March 1940)
3. Hitler's Account of His Own Infancy (1926)
4. Shakespeare's Sonnets
5. Lenny's Dialogues 11 September and 11 November 1991

APPENDIX 1

Supporting References

A. Papers

Johnson, B (2022a), 'Emotional Dwarfism' is a Failure to Thrive Emotionally—Whence the Childhood Roots of Hate, Psychosis, Violence, and Nucleargeddon—All Curable. https://www.davidpublisher.com/Public/uploads/Contribute/621598ee23d5d.pdf (free).

Johnson, B (2022b), Hitler's 'Hate-Syndrome' Proves that All Hatred is Hollow (doi: 10.17265/2159-5313/2022.04.006). https://www.davidpublisher.com/Public/uploads/Contribute/626b6125964a9.pdf (free).

Johnson, B (2021a), Psychiatry is Bereft—It Lacks a Workable Philosophy for Consciousness—Herewith a Three Pronged Escape Plan, *Philosophy Study*, November 2021, Vol. 11, No. 11: 797–809. https://www.davidpublisher.com/Public/uploads/Contribute/619f0119e0b56.pdf (free).

Johnson, B (2021b), The Simple Science of Psychiatry, Psychodrugs and of WAR—Friendless Childhoods Foment Warring Adults, *Philosophy Study*, August 2021, Vol. 11, No. 8: 577–599 (doi: 10.17265/2159-5313/2021.08.001). https://www.davidpublisher.com/Public/uploads/Contribute/61147956e7f0f.pdf (free).

Johnson, B (2021c), The Simple Science of Democracy and of Money—Without Consent, We're Extinct, *Philosophy Study*, 11(5): 311–326 (doi:10.17265/2159-5313/2020.06.003). https://www.davidpublisher.com/Public/uploads/Contribute/60ac4a3a5623c.pdf (free).

Johnson, B (2021d), Why Dysfunctional Medical Flaws Have Cramped Psychiatrists Since 1980, *Journal of US-China Medical Science*, 18: 99–105 (doi:10.17265/1548-6648/2021.03.001): https://www.davidpublisher.com/Public/uploads/Contribute/617f83e4ef9c5.pdf (free).

Johnson, B (2020a), The Simple Science of Sanity, Certainty, and Peace-of-Mind—Empowering 'Intent' Detoxifies Psychosis: https://www.davidpublisher.com/Public/uploads/Contribute/5f7fbbfa4e4ce.pdf (free).

Johnson, B (2020b), The Scientific Basis for Democracy, Peace, Enemies and War—Without 'Intent', We're Fossils, *Philosophy Study*, 10(8): 472–491. (doi:10.17265/2159-5313/2020.08.002). https://www.davidpublisher.com/Public/uploads/Contribute/5f3f7f1ada86d.pdf (free).

Johnson, B (2020c), The Scientific Evidence that Artificial Intelligence (AI) will Continue to Fail, Until We Deploy 'Intent', *Sociology Study*, 10(2): 92–102. (doi:10.17265/2159-5526/2020.02.006). https://www.davidpublisher.com/Public/uploads/Contribute/5f179ecae9a01.pdf (free).

Johnson, B (2020d), The Scientific Evidence that Today's Psychiatry Cripples Itself—By Excluding Intent, *Philosophy Study*, 10(6): 347–359 (doi: 10.17265/2159-5313/2020.06.003). https://www.davidpublisher.com/Public/uploads/Contribute/5eec5e333dc4f.pdf (free).

Johnson, B, (2020e), Why Quakerism is More Scientific than Einstein, *Philosophy Study*, 10(4): 233–251. (doi:10.17265/2159-5313/2020.04.002). https://www.davidpublisher.com/Public/uploads/Contribute/5e9ecb0b231e3.pdf (free).

Johnson, B (2019), Our Midas Disease—Curing Our Money Addiction (unpublished).

Johnson, B (2017), The Scientific Evidence that 'Intent' is Vital for Healthcare, *Open Journal of Philosophy*, 7: 422–434. https://www.scirp.org/journal/paperinformation.aspx?paperid=79128

Johnson, B (2016), Consciousness: Using Clinical Evidence to Link Consciousness with its Twin Perils of Psychosis and Violence. In L Alvarado (ed.), *Consciousness: Social Perspectives, Psychological Approaches and Current Research*, New York: Nova Science Publishers Inc.

Johnson, B (2011), Consciousness Reinstated Using the Certainty Principle—A Better Mental Health Strategy, *Nutrition and Health*, 20(3-4): 183–195.

Johnson, R A (Bob) (1986), Adverse Reactions in Ten Years' General Practice, Computer Analysed, *Journal of the Royal Society of Medicine*, 79(3): 145–148. Retrieved from https://www.ncbi.nlm.nih.gov/pmc/articles/PMC1290232/

Johnson, R A (Bob) (1980), Real Time Retrieval of Clinical Data (PhD Thesis, UMIST, UK). Retrieved from https://www.librarysearch.manchester.ac.uk/discovery/fulldisplay?docid=alma9929780861658016318&context=L&vid=44MAN_INST:MU_NUI&lang=en&search_scope=MyInst_and_CI&adaptor=Local%20Search%20Engine&isFrbr=true&tab=Everythin g&query=any,contains,Real%20time%20retrieval%20of%20clinical%20

data&sortby=date_d&facet=frbrgroupid,include,48412289304630989&offset=0& pcAvailability=false

Johnson, R A (Bob) (1974), A Method of Evaluating Treatment in General Practice, *Journal of the Royal College of General Practitioners*, 24(149): 832–836. Retrieved from https://www.ncbi.nlm.nih.gov/pubmed/4461818

Johnson, R A (Bob) (1972), Computer Analysis of the Complete Medical Record, Including Symptoms and Treatment, *Journal of the Royal College of General Practitioners*, 22(123): 655–660. Retrieved from https://www.ncbi.nlm.nih.gov/ pmc/ articles/PMC2156940/

B. Books

Johnson, B (2018), *How Verbal Physiotherapy Works, Using Social Delight to Defeat Social Harm, For All*, Trust Consent Publishing: www.smashwords.com/books/ view/892956

(2006), *Unsafe at Any Dose — Exposing Psychiatric Dogmas — So Minds Can Heal*, Trust Consent Publishing: www.amazon.co.uk/ unsafe-any-dose-exposing-psychiatric-ebook/dp/B004R9Q5ZY/

(2005) (2 edn.), *Emotional Health, What Emotions Are and How They Cause Social and Mental Diseases*, Trust Consent Publishing: www.smashwords.com/ books/900085

C. Videos

Professor Bob Johnson, Inaugural Lecture, University of Bolton (2023), Using Warmer Emotions to Melt Past Traumas: www.youtube.com/watch?v=t0JVmuJSu3M

Dr Bob Johnson, Keynote for One Small Thing (2021): www.youtube.com/watch?v=3VbCf0f57As

Bob Johnson — Verbal Physiotherapy - Dispuk - CPH (2019): www.youtube.com/watch?v=vwAv2_wucdM

Lenny's video — Lenny Sept & Nov 1991 SD 480p: www.youtube.com/watch?v=TPaPwBXqe7Y

George Orwell's Review of *Mein Kampf* (1940)

---

§1. It is a sign of the speed at which events are moving that Hurst and Blackett's unexpurgated edition of *Mein Kampf,* published only a year ago, is edited from a pro-Hitler angle. The obvious intention of the translator's preface and notes is to tone down the book's ferocity and present Hitler in as kindly a light as possible. For at that date Hitler was still respectable. He had crushed the German labour movement, and for that the property-owning classes were willing to forgive him almost anything. Both Left and Right concurred in the very shallow notion that National Socialism was merely a version of Conservatism.

§2. Then suddenly it turned out that Hitler was not respectable after all. As one result of this, Hurst and Blackett's edition was reissued in a new jacket explaining that all profits would be devoted to the Red Cross. Nevertheless, simply on the internal evidence of *Mein Kampf,* **it is difficult to believe that any real change has taken place in Hitler's aims and opinions**. When one compares his utterances of a year or so ago with those made fifteen years earlier, a thing that strikes one is the rigidity of his mind, the way in which **his world-view doesn't develop**.

§3. It is the fixed vision of a monomaniac and not likely to be much affected by the temporary manoeuvres of power politics. Probably, in Hitler's own mind, the Russo-German Pact represents no more than an alteration of time-table. The plan laid down in *Mein Kampf* was to smash Russia first, with the implied intention of smashing England afterwards. Now, as it has turned out, England has got to be dealt with first, because Russia was the more easily bribed of the two. But Russia's turn will come when England is out of the picture — that, no doubt, is how Hitler sees it. Whether it will turn out that way is of course a different question.

§4. Suppose that Hitler's programme could be put into effect. What he envisages, a hundred years hence, is a continuous state of 250 million Germans with plenty of 'living room' (i.e. stretching to Afghanistan or thereabouts), **a horrible brainless empire** in which, essentially, nothing ever happens except the training of young men for war and the endless breeding of fresh cannon-fodder.

§5. How was it that he was able to put this monstrous vision across? It is easy to say that at one stage of his career he was financed by the heavy industrialists, who saw in him the man who would smash the Socialists and Communists. They would not have backed him, however, if he had not talked a great movement into existence already. Again, the situation in Germany, with its seven million unemployed, was obviously favourable for demagogues. But Hitler could not have succeeded against his many rivals if it had not been for **the attraction of his own personality,** which one can feel even in the clumsy writing of *Mein Kampf,* and which is no doubt overwhelming when one hears his speeches.

§6. The fact is that there is something deeply appealing about him. One feels it again when one sees his photographs—and I recommend especially the photograph at the beginning of Hurst and Blackett's edition, which shows Hitler in his early Brownshirt days. It is a pathetic, dog-like face, the face of **a man suffering under intolerable wrongs.** In a rather more manly way it reproduces the expression of innumerable pictures of Christ crucified, and there is little doubt that that is how Hitler sees himself.

§7. **The initial, personal cause of his grievance against the universe can only be guessed at;** but at any rate the grievance is here. He is the martyr, the victim, Prometheus chained to the rock, the self-sacrificing hero who fights single-handed against impossible odds. If he were killing a mouse he would know how to make it seem like a dragon. One feels, as with Napoleon, that he is fighting against destiny, that he can't win, and yet that he somehow deserves to. The attraction of such a pose is of course enormous; **half the films that one sees turn upon some such theme.**

§8. Also he has grasped the falsity of the hedonistic attitude to life. Nearly all western thought since the last war, certainly all 'progressive' thought, has assumed tacitly that human beings desire nothing beyond **ease, security and avoidance of pain.** In such a view of life there is no room, for instance, for patriotism and the military virtues. The Socialist who finds his children playing with soldiers is usually upset, but he is never able to think of a substitute for the tin soldiers; tin pacifists somehow won't do.

§9. Hitler, **because in his own joyless mind he feels it with exceptional strength,** knows that human beings don't only want comfort, safety, short working-hours, hygiene, birth-control and, in general, common sense; they also, at least intermittently, want struggle and self-sacrifice, not to mention drums, flags and loyalty-parades. However they may be as economic theories, Fascism and Nazism are psychologically far sounder than any hedonistic conception of life. The same is probably true of Stalin's militarised version of Socialism. All three of the great dictators have enhanced their power by imposing intolerable burdens on their peoples. Whereas Socialism, and even capitalism in a more grudging way, have said to people 'I offer you a good time,' Hitler has said to them 'I offer you struggle, danger and death,' and as a result a whole nation flings itself at his feet. Perhaps later on they will get sick of it and change their minds, as at the end of the last war.

§10. After a few years of slaughter and starvation 'Greatest happiness of the greatest number' is a good slogan, but at this moment 'Better an end with horror than a horror without end' is a winner. Now that we are fighting against the man who coined it, we ought not to underrate its emotional appeal.

Written in March 1940

Reference: https://carnegiecouncil-media.storage.googleapis.com/files/v18_i007-008_a010.pdf

From *The Collected Essays, Journalism and Letters of George Orwell*, Volume 2, edited by Sonia Orwell and Ian Angus, copyright 1968 by Sonia Brownell Orwell. Reprinted by permission of Harcourt Brace Jovanovich, Inc. Paragraph numbers and emphases added.

APPENDIX 3

Hitler's Account of His Own Infancy (1926)

§1. Here is an example: in a basement consisting of two stuffy rooms lives a labourer's family of seven. Among the five children is a boy of three years. This is the age when a child first becomes conscious of things around him. Gifted people carry memories of that period far into old age.

§2. The small, overcrowded space produces an unfortunate situation. The conditions often generate quarrels and bickering. The people are not living with one another; they are merely living in the same place, squeezed together. Every small argument leads to a sickening quarrel. In a larger dwelling, the argument would be easily smoothed out simply by separation. The children may tolerate these conditions because children can quarrel constantly and forget the argument quickly. However, a daily battle between parents slowly teaches the children a lesson. The dispute may take the form of a father's brutality to a mother, of drunken maltreatment. Any person who does not know of this life can hardly imagine it. By the time the boy goes from three to six, he has developed a working idea of the world which must horrify even an adult. Now, he is morally infected and physically undernourished, and the young 'citizen' is sent to primary school with vermin living in his poor little scalp.

§3. Now, with great difficulty, he must learn reading and writing, and that is about all he can manage.

§4. Studying at home is out of the question. Father and mother argue and use language that would not be socially appropriate right in front of their own children, making studying impossible. But when the parents talk to teachers and school officials, they are more inclined to talk roughly to them than to turn their young child over their knee and introduce him to reason. Nothing the little fellow hears at home strengthens his respect for his fellow human beings. [*Was der kleine Kerl sonst noch alles zu Hause hört, führt auch nicht zu einer Stärkung der Achtung vor der lieben Mitwelt.*]

§5. They never utter a good word about humanity. No institution is safe from their profane attacks, from the school teacher to the head of the state. No matter whether it is religion or morals, state or society, everything is defamed and dragged in the muck. When the boy leaves school at the age of fourteen, it is hard to tell which is greater—his incredible stupidity where common knowledge and basic skills are concerned, or his biting disrespect and bad manners.

§6. The immoral displays, even at that age, make one's hair stand on end. [*Auftretens verbunden mit einer Unmoral schon in diesem Alter, daß einem die Haare zu Berge stehen könnten.*]

§7. He holds almost nothing sacred. He has never met true greatness, but he has experienced the abyss of everyday life. What position can he possibly occupy in the world which he is about to enter? The three-year-old child has become a fifteen-year-old who despises all authority. Aside from filth and uncleanliness, he has yet to find anything which might stir him to any high enthusiasm.

§8. As he begins the more demanding parts of his life, he falls into the ruts he has learned from his father. He wanders about, comes home Heaven knows when, beats the tattered creature who was once his mother, curses God and the world, and finally he is sentenced to a prison for juvenile delinquents.

§9. Here, he gets his final polish.

Mein Kampf (1926), Chapter 2, p.24. Paragraph numbers added.

APPENDIX 4

Shakespeare Sonnets

Sonnet 116

Let me not to the marriage of true minds
Admit impediments, love is not love
Which alters when it alteration finds,
Or bends with the remover to remove.
O no, it is an ever-fixéd mark
That looks on tempests and is never shaken;
It is the star to every wand'ring bark,
Whose worth's unknown, although his height be taken.
Love's not Time's fool, though rosy lips and cheeks
Within his bending sickle's compass come,
Love alters not with his brief hours and weeks,
But bears it out even to the edge of doom:
If this be error and upon me proved,
I never writ, nor no man ever loved.

Sonnet 18

Shall I compare thee to a summer's day?
Thou art more lively[1] and more temperate:
Rough winds do shake the darling buds of May,
And summer's lease hath all too short a date:
Sometime too hot the eye of heaven shines,
And often is his gold complexion dimmed,
And every fair from fair sometime declines,
By chance, or nature's changing course untrimmed:

---

1. For the correct use of 'lively' rather than 'lovely', see Padel, J (1981), *New Poems by Shakespeare: Order and Meaning Restored to the Sonnets*, New Mermaids.

But thy eternal summer shall not fade,
Nor lose possession of that fair thou ow'st,
Nor shall death brag thou wand'rest in his shade,
When in eternal lines to time thou grow'st,
So long as men can breathe or eyes can see,
So long lives this, and this gives life to thee.

APPENDIX 5

Lenny's Dialogues 11 September and 11 November 1991

11 September 1991

Line

1. Bob: How would you describe to someone who doesn't know anything about it, what questions I am asking you and what we are doing?

2. Lenny: Well it's about my Mother, how she used to batter me when I was a kid.

3. B: What effect did this have on you?

4. L: Well it made me frightened.

5. B: Did it?

6. L: Yes.

7. B: What's happened to the fear?

8. L: It's embedded.

9. B: It's still there is it?

10. L: Yes.

11. B: It doesn't help you does it?

12. L: No.

13. B: What effect does this embedded fear have?

14. L: It's made me violent.

15. B: Did it?

16. L: Yes.

17. B: How does that work?

18. L: I don't know.

19. B: Why does embedded fear make you violent?

20.   L: Well she used violence on me all the time and I grew up to violence didn't I? Do you know what I mean?

21.   B: But you're a big lad and you're an adult so why are you still frightened of your Mother? It's still there isn't it?

22.   L: I'm still there, yes.

23.   B: So why hasn't it changed. Why is it still there, do you think?

24.   L: Well, it's all part of growing up isn't it?

25.   B: Part of you hasn't has it?

26.   L: Yes.

27.   B: Part of you is still there, isn't it?

28.   L: Yes.

29.   B: Because we talked about that this morning didn't we?

30.   L: Yes.

31.   B: Being an adult. Can you tell her you're an adult?

32.   L: Yes, I could try.

33.   B: Would you find it difficult?

34.   L: Yes.

35.   B: You would, wouldn't you?

36.   L: Yes.

37.   B: Do you find that surprising, that you find it difficult to tell your mother you're an adult?

38.   L: Yes. Very surprising.

39.   B: It is isn't it? So what will stop you? Say your mother was sitting over there, what would you say to her?

40.   L: I'd say 'Mother you can't hit me any more. I am an adult.'

41.   B: And you believe that?

42.   L: Yes, partly.

43.   B: You partly believe it and partly don't?

44.   L: Yes. I don't know whether I could say it to her or not.

45.   B: What would stop you?

46.   L: Fear.

47.   B: Fear of what? What is she going to do?

48.   L: Well she might get up and clout me.

49.   B: Might she?

50.   L: Well she might.

51. B: How old is she?
52. L: 85.
53. B: And she is going to do you an injury is she?
54. L: Oh she's still lively.
55. B: 85. How big is she?
56. L: 5 feet 2 inches.
57. B: And how big are you?
58. L: 6 feet 3½ inches.
59. B: It doesn't sound much of a match does it?
60. L: No, but you can't hit a woman can you?
61. B: You can't disagree with your Mother, let alone hit her can you?
62. L: No.
63. B: Do you need to be able to disagree with her?
64. L: It would be nice to, wouldn't it?
65. B: Would it? What advantage to you is disagreeing with your Mother?
66. L: Well, I could get on with my own life.
67. B: Could you?
68. L: Yes.
69. B: What would you tell her?
70. L: I'd say leave me alone.
71. B: Get out of my life?
72. L: That's why I left home.
73. B: Why did you leave home?
74. L: Because I couldn't put up with her batterings any more.
75. B: You couldn't, could you?
76. L: No.
77. B: How old were you when you left home?
78. L: Oh don't forget I was in Approved School so I left when I was 13 and I didn't go back home. Oh I'm a liar, I did go back home, I did, but it was getting on my nerves, all the shouting and bawling.
79. B: And even at that time you were still afraid of your Mother weren't you?
80. L: Oh yes.
81. B: You said this morning you were programmed. What was the programme?

82.   L: Programmed to be afraid of my mother.

83.   B: You were weren't you?

84.   L: Yes.

85.   B: Also programmed to be smaller than her.

86.   L: Yes, she thinks I am still in shorts.

87.   B: She does doesn't she?

88.   L: She does.

89.   B: So are you going to tell her? ... I beg your pardon?

90.   B: Are you going to tell her?

91.   L: If she was here now.

92.   B: Yes.

93.   L: If she was here now — and if you was here.

94.   B: Right.

95.   L: Mother you can't touch me I'm an adult. I would, I would say that.

96.   B: You would?

97.   L: Yes.

98.   B: That's because I'm here?

99.   L: That's because you're here.

100.   B: What role do I play? How am I helping you to do that?

101.   L: Well, you are giving me ... power.

102.   B: Moral support?

103.   L: Yes.

104.   B: I am aren't I?

105.   L: Yes.

106.   B: After a while you can do it for yourself without me can't you?

107.   L: Oh, of course, yes.

108.   B: But at the moment you need my support.

109.   L: Yes.

110.   B: Which I am very happy to give you because I believe you are an adult and I believe she should be told. [Both laugh] That's right isn't it?

111.   L: Yes.

112.   B: Now could you tell me something about your violence and how that relates to fear of your Mother, if it does.

113.   L: I've been pushed around and pushed around and pushed around that much, that I just couldn't take any more when this lad started, and I just went too far.
114.   B: How does that relate to your Mother?
115.   L: Well, it's bound to isn't it?
116.   B: Go on then.
117.   L: She used violence on me and I couldn't do anything back.
118.   B: You couldn't do anything back.
119.   L: No, and when he started giving me some lip...
120.   B: Right.
121.   L: I battered the hell out of him.
122.   B: Yes.
123.   L: And I've got to say it: I meant to kill him.
124.   B: You did?
125.   L: I did.
126.   B: How does that relate to ...?
127.   L: There's no getting away from it. As I was saying to the policeman 'I want to kill you, you bastard', and I killed him — That's why I wish I hadn't gone for diminished responsibility.
128.   B: What does that mean?
129.   L: Manslaughter.
130.   B: That's what you went for?
131.   L: Yes, I should have just pleaded guilty to murder, maybe I wouldn't have been on the Book [Category A].
132.   B: So how is that violence related to fear of your Mother? How does that work?
133.   L: Have you never heard of this before? If violence is shown to you time and time again, there comes a time in your life when you just snap, and I snapped.
134.   B: Right.
135.   L: Do you get the point?
136.   B: I do.
137.   L: So you can say it's down to her.
138.   B: Because of the violence coming from her?
139.   L: Yes because of the violence coming from her.

140. B: And what's your defence against the violence coming from her
      again?

141. L: No chance.

142. B: What are you going to do. How are you going to stop it?

143. L: I'm going to tell her.

144. B: What are you going to tell her?

145. L: That I'm an adult.

146. B: You like that don't you?

147. L: Yes.

148. B: You're getting stronger as you say it, aren't you?

149. L: Yes, I am.

150. B: You can feel yourself getting more confident.

151. L: I'm getting angry as well.

152. B: Are you, with her?

153. L: With her.

154. B: You are, aren't you? You see the anger. I agree with you, the anger
      and violence can live together, but behind the anger is fear,
      because you feel that there is no defence against your Mother
      doing it again.

155. L: She'd never be able to do it again.

156. B: I know that.

157. L: I know that.

158. B: That's it.

159. L: I know that.

160. B: You also know you're an adult, don't you?

161. L: Yes.

162. B: And you can tell her that?

163. L: Yes I can do.

164. B: At the moment with assistance from me. But in due course on
      your own.

165. L: On my own, yes.

166. B: That's right. Look her straight in the eye and say 'Look Ma I'm an
      adult'. Can you do that?

167. L: Yes.

168. B: Go on then.

169. L: Look Ma, I am an adult. And you can't touch me ever again. I've grown up, I haven't still got shorts on.
170. B: Does that give you confidence?
171. L: Yes it does, saying it.
172. B: Does it calm your anger down?
173. L: Yes it does, yes.
174. B: Does it?
175. L: Yes it does.
176. B: It gives a way out for it, doesn't it?
177. L: Yes.
178. B: Because that's the reality.
179. L: Course it is, yes.
180. B: So is this helping you, would you say?
181. L: Yes, it is helping me.
182. B: How would you summarise your position and how have I been able to help you?
183. L: Well, nobody's ever bothered before. They've just asked a few questions and that's it—blah blah blah thank you mam and all that rubbish. The psychologist doesn't do anything.
184. B: So what questions have I asked you? And what has been helpful?
185. L: Well, you have asked me what my home life was like. Why did I start getting into trouble?
186. B: You've got an explanation for that now, haven't you?
187. L: Yes.
188. B: Which you can work out for yourself now, as it were.
189. L: Yes, that's right.
190. B: You've done very well. So you will get rid of this fear in due course?
191. L: Yes, I will.
192. B: How big is it this fear?
193. L: Not all that big now.
194. B: It was big before?
195. L: It was big when you started.
196. B: Was it?
197. L: Yes.

198.   B: What did you think when I first started questioning you in this area?

199.   L: I thought you was a 'quack' [both laugh].

200.   B: Did you believe what I was saying?

201.   L: I did but I wanted to shy away from the truth.

202.   B: Did you?

203.   L: But I told you the truth didn't I? I have told you the truth.

204.   B: Certainly.

205.   L: I could have said 'Ah well I don't want nowt to do with it' and walked off, couldn't I?

206.   B: Yes.

207.   L: It's like coming up against a brick wall isn't it?

208.   B: People do that.

209.   L: Yes, they shouldn't do that.

210.   B: So you were going to do that to begin with?

211.   L: I was going to do, yes.

212.   B: What was wrong? What was going to make you do that?

213.   L: It was upsetting me — the way you was going on about it.

214.   B: Was it?

215.   L: Yes.

216.   B: What exactly upset you?

217.   L: Against my Mother.

218.   B: You didn't like that at all?

219.   L: No.

220.   B: That's right.

221.   L: But I had to go with it because it was the truth.

222.   B: Because what I think that goes wrong is, because I frighten people by going at it too much to begin with. Is that what you think, would you agree that?

223.   L: When you kept saying about the spanners.

224.   B: You've got the old pliers and pincers didn't you?

225.   L: Yes, that's true.

226.   B: But you stuck with it, didn't you?

227.   L: Yes I did, yes.

228. B: You did very well. But you fancied stopping it at the beginning did you?
229. L: Yes, I did.
230. B: Because it was getting a bit near the bone?
231. L: That's right yes, but it's the truth, isn't it? The truth's got to come out hasn't it? And you were trying to help me, and I am helping you.
232. B: I'm sure you are. So when the truth comes out what would you say the truth was, that's got to come out.
233. L: Well the truth's got to come out and say right I'm not scared of my Mother any more. I'm going to tell her outright, I'm an adult, no joking about. And say look, I've grown up now, you have got to start talking nice, and all that, no shouting like you normally do.
234. B: And no threatening to batter you like she does.
235. L: Yes, that's right.
236. B: So the fear of her will disappear.
237. L: Yes.
238. B: Can you see how your anger went down. A little earlier on you were saying that you were angry, but the anger went down when you understood where it was coming from.
239. L: That's true yes, it's very true.
240. B: And that's the secret isn't it?
241. L: Yes.
242. B: Magic. Anyway thanks for coming along. And let me just double check that you don't mind if I show this to different people.
243. L: No, I don't mind at all.
244. B: Thank you very much indeed.
245. L: All right Bob.
246. B: Thanks, see you.
247. L: See you.

11 November 1991 — Extract

248. L: You can't hit your own mother. Whenever she battered me, I'd never dream of lifting a hand to hit her. Even when I was 21, she slapped me across the face. And me Dad came in. And I ran out

of the house. And slammed the door, and then just went and got pissed.

249.   B: And bottled it up.

250.   L: Yes.

251.   B: But now you would stop her, if she came to hit you?

252.   L: There's no way she would hit me now.

253.   B: What would you say?

254.   L: I wouldn't have to say anything — if she went to slap me, I'd just hold her hand. [Both laugh]

255.   B: well you didn't have the confidence to do that before.

256.   L: If this had've happened years ago, where a doctor had taken an interest say when I was in my twenties and said what you'd said and we'd conquered it, [none of this would have happened].

257.   And then I went to the house. And say I came in late, and she said blah blah blah and she went to hit me, I'd say mother you can't hit me love — I'm a grown up. You can't do it. You can kick me out of the house.

258.   B: Because it's your house.

259.   L: But you can't hit me — don't try and hit me.

260.   B: But you've never said that up until the last month or two.

261.   L: Yes. I've never had the confidence to say it.

262.   B: That's right.

263.   L: You're brain washed into fear … [continued].

All the above from the author's professional notes made/transcribed at the time. See also Lenny's video in *Appendix 1*, Supporting References, C. Videos.

Index

Danger, Development and Adaptation

Seminal Papers on the Dynamic-Maturational Model of Attachment and Adaptation

Patricia McKinsey Crittenden, Foreword by Rodolfo de Bernart

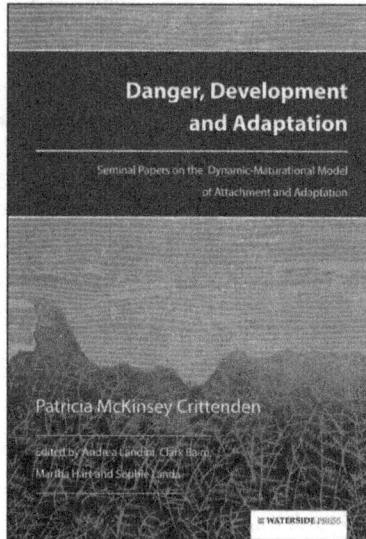

Edited by Andrea Landini, Martha Hart, Clark Baim and Sophie Landa.

In association with the International Association for the Study of Attachment.

'Thought-provoking and insightful.'
Dante Cicchetti, Professor of Child Psychology and Psychiatry,
Institute of Child Development, University of Minnesota

Hardback and paperback
ISBN 978-1-909976-27-6 | 2015

Parenting and Child Development

Issues and Answers

Dr Nicole Letourneau

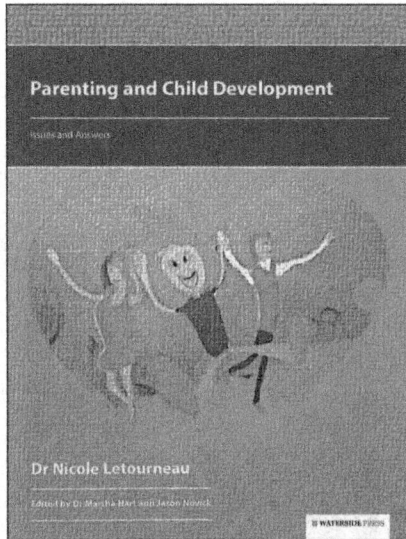

Edited by Dr Martha Hart and Jason Novick.

Essential reading for anyone and everyone wanting to improve mother-child interaction and child developmental outcomes including in cases of high-risk.

Hardback, paperback & ebook

ISBN 978-1-909976-77-1 | 2020

www.WatersidePress.co.uk

The Prison Psychiatrist's Wife

Sue Johnson

Foreword Charles Bronson

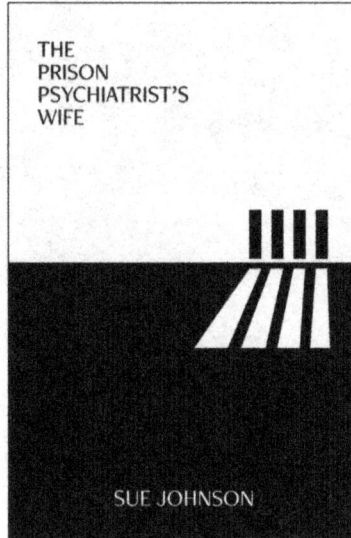

A gripping true story of a Herculean project as Sue Johnson's psychiatrist husband Bob, recruited to work with notorious offenders at Parkhurst Prison, sets out to discover whether he can change dangerous and violent men.

'A tremendous book. A perspective that needs to be heard.'
Oliver James, Author, Broadcaster and Clinical Psychologist

'A rollercoaster ride of emotion, courage, and political chicanery … I was held by the power of the narrative.'
Dave Marteau, former Head of HM Prison Drug Addiction Service

'This is phenomenology… women's writing like Virginia Woolf.'
Professor Emerita Eleanor Godway, Central Connecticut State University

Paperback & ebook | ISBN 978-1-914603-30-3 | 2023